HYPERCALCEMIA PATHOPHYSIOLOGY & TREATMENT

By

Franco Lumachi & Stefano M.M. Basso

CONTENTS

FOREWORD

Changes in serum calcium concentration regulate several fundamental cellular events, including enzymatic activities, and cell membranes excitability. In adults 99% of calcium is found in the skeleton, in which it plays both structural and regulatory roles. High blood calcium levels (hypercalcemia) is extremely rare under physiological conditions. It usually occurs when parathyroid hormone (PTH) and 1,25 (OH)$_2$ vitamin D act on osteocytic osteolysis and osteoclastic resorption, transferring calcium to the extracellular compartment. Basic mechanisms regulating calcium metabolism have long been defined, but the complete role of new factors, such as fibroblast growth factor-23 (FGF-23), transient receptor potential cation channel, subfamily V member 5 (TRPV5), and the Klotho gene, is still under study. The main causes of hypercalcemia are primary hyperparathyroidism (HPT), and malignancy-associated hypercalcemia (MAH). Severe or prolonged hypercalcemia may cause several complications, mainly depending on serum calcium concentrations. In any case, the clinical features are usually aspecific, such as muscle weakness, fatigability, asthenia, as well as signs and symptoms of dehydration. Other less common causes of hypercalcemia include increased intake of calcium and vitamin D, granulomatous diseases, other endocrine disorders, multiple endocrine neoplasia, familial benign hypocalciuric hypocalcemia, and other rare disorders.

The therapy of choice for HPT is the surgical ablation of the hyperfunctioning parathyroid tissue, and the best time to cure a patient is during the initial phase. In patients with primary HPT, parathyroidectomy produces a sudden modification of the endocrine balance which regulates the calcium and phosphate metabolism. Currently, minimally invasive parathyroidectomy is widely performed, both videoassisted and radioguided. Physiologically, PTH acts directly on the renal and bone cells, and indirectly it influences the intestinal absorption of calcium, stimulating the renal synthesis of $[1,25(OH)_2]D_3$. Although there is an immediate renal response to serum PTH levels, The modifications which take place in the bone are slower, according to the particular way of the bone-remodeling process. The antireabsorptive action of bisphopshonates has been considered the most effective in the disorders characterized by an excessive bone resorption. Unfortunately, patients with MAH have usually advanced tumors which explains short survival rate. However, when the first diagnosis is a chemosensitive tumor, such as multiple myeloma or metastatic breast cancer, long-term remissions may be obtained. Calicimimetic drugs and humanized monoclonal antibody against human parathyroid hormone-related protein represent the new drugs useful to treat hypercalcemia.

Serum calcium has a pivotal role in the homeostasis of an organism, and its alteration has important effects. Knowledge of role and regulatory mechanisms of serum calcium is crucial to understand and diagnose the underlying diseases, that cause hypercalcemia. This book is a compilation of the efforts of a selected group of well-established experts in the field of calcium metabolism, and management of the causes of hypercalcemia. It summarizes the principle findings and points out possible pitfalls in hypercalcemic diseases, with the aim to help both students in the understanding and clinicians in their approach to patients with hypercalcemia.

We would like to thank Director Mahmood Alam and particularly Assistant Manager Asma Ahmed, together with the whole Bentham Science Publishers, for their effort and support.

Franco Lumachi, M.D.
Associate Professor of Surgery
University of Padua, School of Medicine
35128 Padova, Italy

Stefano M.M. Basso, M.D., Ph.D.
Assistant Professor
S. Maria degli Angeli Hospital
33170 Pordenone, Italy

PREFACE

Hypercalcemia is a relatively common disorder, which requires specific treatment in order to control symptoms and prevent the development of organ damage. Since primary hyperparathyroidism and malignancy are responsible for more than 90% of all cases of hypercalcemia, greater interest was given in terms of developing the best strategy to manage these two critical situations.

The aim of this book is to present up-to-date knowledge on hypercalcemia, its association with renal disorders, and benign and malignant diseases, diagnostic methodologies, as well as surgical and medical treatment. Insights into the etiology, pathogenesis and pathophysiology of hypercalcemia are included in the first four chapters, also providing comprehensive descriptions of clinical features, diagnostic and treatment procedures in the specific diseases associated with hypercalcemia.

The other chapters present details on biochemical findings and ways to monitor complications and therapy, giving suggestions on the current imaging techniques, and deal with the criteria, procedures and results of surgical treatment of hypercalcemia, including unilateral and minimally-invasive parathyroidectomy. Finally, a specific chapter describes the pharmacology of anti-hypercalcemic drugs, also providing information on new drugs and future perspectives.

Uniquely, this book will serve as a complete reference source for oncologists, nephrologists, endocrinologists and other clinicians, as well as for biochemists and pharmacologists, and all those involved in hypercalcemia management and research.

John G. Delinassios
Director
International Institute of Anticancer Research
Athens, Greece

CONTRIBUTORS

Stefano M.M. Basso, M.D., Ph.D.
Assistant Professor, Division of Surgery I
S.M. degli Angeli Hospital, 33170 Pordenone, Italy

Umberto Basso, M.D.
Assistant Professor, Istituto Oncologico Veneto (IOV), IRCCS, 35128 Padova, Italy

Antonella Brunello, M.D.
Clinical Research Assistant, Istituto Oncologico Veneto (IOV), IRCCS, 35128 Padova, Italy

Valentina Camozzi, M.D., Ph.D.
Clinical Research, Department of Medical & Surgical Sciences
University of Padua, School of Medicine, 35128 Padova, Italy

Piero Cappelletti, M.D.
Assistant professor, Director, Department of Clinical Pathology
S. Maria degli Angeli Hospital, 33170 Pordenone, Italy

Gianpietro Feltrin, M.D.
Professor, Director, Radiology Section, Department of Diagnostic Medical Sciences
University of Padua, School of Medicine, 35128 Padova, Italy

Chiara Franzin, Ph.D.
Research Associate, Department of Medical & Surgical Sciences
University of Padua, School of Medicine, 35128 Padova, Italy

Grazia Guzzetta, M.D.
Radiology Resident, Department of Diagnostic Medical Sciences
University of Padua, School of Medicine, 35128 Padova, Italy

Maria Guzzetta, M.D.
Radiology Resident, Department of Diagnostic Medical Sciences
University of Padua, School of Medicine, 35128 Padova, Italy

Giovanni Luisetto, M.D.
Associate Professor of Internal Medicine, Department of Medical & Surgical Sciences
University of Padua, School of Medicine, 35128 Padova, Italy

Franco Lumachi, M.D.
Associate Professor of Surgery, Department of Surgical & Gastroenterological Sciences
University of Padua, School of Medicine, 35128 Padova, Italy

Walter Mancini, M.D.
Assistant Professor, Director, Division of Nephrology
S. Maria degli Angeli Hospital, 33170 Pordenone, Italy

Fabiana Nascimben, M.D.
Clinical Research, Emergency Department
S. Maria degli Angeli Hospital, 33170 Pordenone, Italy

Anna Roma, M.D.
Medical Oncology Resident, Istituto Oncologico Veneto (IOV), IRCCS, 35128 Padova, Italy

Renato Tozzoli, M.D.
Assistant Professor, Director, Department of Clinical Chemistry & Microbiology
City Hospital, 33053 Latisana, Italy

ACRONYMS USED IN THIS BOOK

AABD	Aluminium-associated bone disease
ABC	Airway-Breathing-Circulation
ABD	Adynamic bone syndrome
ACLS	Advanced Cardiac Life Support
ADH	Antidiuretic hormone
ALP	Alkaline phosphatise
AMG-26	Denosumab
ANK	Ankyrin
ATP	Adenosine triphosphate
BAP	Bone alkaline phosphatise
BMD	Bone mineral density
BNE	Bilateral neck exploration
BSA	Body surface area
CASR	Calcium-sensing receptor
CDKN	Cyclin-dependent kinase inhibitor
CDKN1B	Cyclin-dependent kinase inhibitor 1B
CKD	Chronic kidney disease
CLIA	Electrochemiluminescens
CN	Cortical nephrocalcinosis
CPK	Creatinphosphokinase
Cr-clearance	Creatinine clearance
CT	Computed tomography
CTx	Collagen cross-link-associated C-telopeptide
CVa	Analytical variation
CVP	Central venous pressure
DKK1	Wingless-type inhibitory Dickkopfs1
DPD	Deoxypyridoline
DXA	Dual-energy x-ray absorptiometry
eGFR	Estimated glomerular filtration rate
ESRD	End stage of renal disease
FBHH	Familial benign hypocalciuric hypercalcemia
FDG	^{18}F-fluoro-2-deoxyglucose
FGF	Fibroblast growth factor
FIPH	Familial isolated primary hyperparathyroidism
FPP	Farnesyl pyrophosphate
FPPS	Farnesyl pyrophosphate synthase
GFR	Glomerular filtration rate
GGPP	Geranylgeranyl pyrophosphate
HAP	Hydroxyapatite
HPLC	High-pressure liquid chromatography
HPT	Hyperparathyroidism
HPT-JT	Hyperparathyroidsim-jaw tumor
HRCT	High-resolution computed tomography
HRPT2	Hyperparathyroidism 2
iCa	Ionozed calcium
IL-1	Interleukin-1
IMAS	Competitive immunoassay
iPTH	Intact parathyroid hormone
IRMA	Immunoradiometric assay
ISE	Ion-selective electrodes
JNK	c-Jung N-terminus kinase

Kf	Filtration coefficient
LC-MS/MS	Liquid chromatography-tandem mass spectrometry
MAH	Malignancy-associated hypercalcemia
MAPK	Mitogen-activated protein thyrosine kinase
MEN	Multiple endocrine neoplasia
MIP	Minimally invasive parathyroidectomy
MN	Medullary nephrocalinosis
MR	Magnetic resonance
N-BPs	Nitrogen bosphosphonates
NF-κ	Nuclear factor -kappa
nN-BPS	Non nitrogen bisphosphonates
NTx	Collagen cross-link-associated N-telopeptide
ONJ	Osteonecrosis of the jaw
OPG	Osteoprotegerin
PBs	Bisphosphonates
PDGFs	Plateled-derived growth factors
PET	Positron emission tomography
PRAD1	Parathyroid adenoma 1
PTH	Parathyroid hormone
PT	Parathyroid
PTHrP	Parathyroid hormone-related protein
PTx	Parathyroidectomy
PYD	Pyridinium cross-links pyridinoline
qPTH	Quick-PTH
QTC	Quantitative computed tomography
RANKL	Receptor activator of nuclear actor-κ ligand
RB	Retinoblastoma
RIA	Radioimmunoassay
RLN	Recurrent laryngeal nerve
SPECT	Single-photon emission computed tomography
TALH	Thick ascending limb of Henle's loop
tCa	Total serum calcium
TGB	Transforming growth factor
TNF	Tumor necrosis factor
TPN	Total parenteral nutrition
TRANCE	TNF-related activation-induced cytokine
TRPV5	Transient receptor potential cation channel, subfamily V member 5
uCa	Urinary calcium
UFCa	Ultrafiltrate calcium
UNE	Unilateral neck exploration
uNTx	Urinary N-telopeptide
US	Ultrasonography
WBS	Whole-body bone scintigraphy
Wnts	Wingless-type

CHAPTER 1

Renal Diseases & Hypercalcemia

Walter Mancini[1], Franco Lumachi[2] and Stefano M.M. Basso[3]

[1]Division of Nephrology, S. Maria degli Angeli Hospital, 33170 Pordenone, Italy; [2]University of Padua, School of Medicine, 35128 Padova, Italy and [3]Division of Surgery I, S. Maria degli Angeli Hospital, 33170 Pordenone, Italy

Abstract: Calcium is the most represented bivalent cation in the organism, and it is essential for a variety of actions. It supports the body, and works as a second messenger, modulating different intracellular and extracellular processes. The balance of parathyroid hormone (PTH), calcitonin, and vitamin D has long been considered the main regulator of calcium metabolism, but the function of other "actors", such as fibroblast growth factor-23 (FGF-23), Klotho gene, and transient receptor potential cation channel, subfamily V, member 5 (TPRV5) should be considered. Hypercalcemia may cause renal damage both temporary (alteration of renal tubular function for instance) and persisting (relapsing nephrolithiasis, especially with high kidney stones) by different ways, leading to a progressive loss of renal function, and ultimately the end stage renal disease with subsequent need of renal replacement therapy. A worsened renal function stimulates further alterations of calcium metabolism, and renal osteodistrophy may result. Hypercalcemia is a common problem also in renal transplant recipients, although in most cases spontaneous resolution occurs, and a modification of the PTH set up, unrelated with extracellular calcium levels, appears very often. In any case, hypercalcemia can lead to alteration of almost the whole renal tubules, modifying the glomerular filtration rate both in direct (vasoconstriction) and indirect (modification of filtration coefficient) ways. Nephrological therapies can treat both acute and chronic hypercalcemia, and it seems to be effective also in secondary hyperparathyroidism (HPT), but in other situations, such as posttransplantation HPT, a surgical approach is often needed.

INTRODUCTION

Calcium is a metallic element essential for normal development and function of the body. It is an important constituent of bones, the matrix of bones consisting principally of calcium phosphate, accounts for about 99% of the body's calcium. Also, it is essential for many metabolic process, including nerve function, muscle contraction, and blood clotting. Hypercalcemia may cause renal impairment, both temporary (alteration of renal tubular function for instance), and progressive (relapsing nephrolithiasis, especially with high kidney stones) by different ways, leading to a progressive loss of renal function, until the end stage of renal disease (ESRD), and the subsequent need of renal replacement therapy.

Hypercalcemia can lead to an alteration of almost the whole renal tubules, modifying the glomerular filtration rate (GFR) both in direct (vasoconstriction) and in indirect (modification of filtration coefficient) ways. This is a common problem also in renal transplant recipients, although in most cases spontaneous resolution occurs. Paradoxically, a worsened renal function stimulates a further alteration of calcium metabolism following different pathways, such as hypocalcemia, reduced renal calcitriol production, reduced expression of receptors for vitamin D and calcium in parathyroid glands. As a result, an alteration of parathyroid hormone (PTH) levels occur, ultimately leading to renal osteodistrophy, which are characterized by different bone features, of which *osteitis fibrosa cystica* is considered the most serious.

Under this condition, an increase of both number and activity of osteoclast is observed, with subsequent decreased bone mineral density (BMD), and fibrotic bone degeneration. However, in the adult healthy subject, both intracellular and extracellular calcium are tightly controlled, and calcium absorbed from the gut passes into various body pools and is lost in the urine (Fig. **1**).

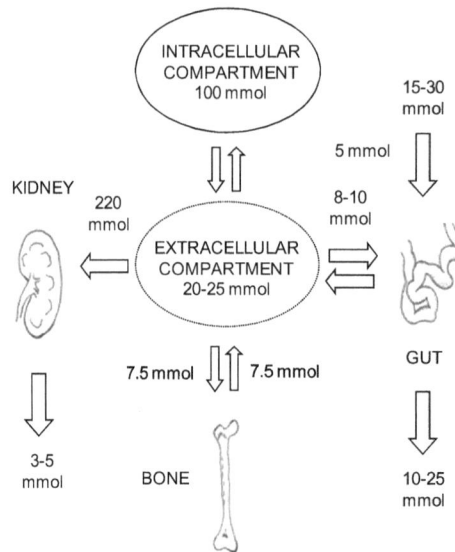

Figure 1: Calcium balance and distribution in healthy adults.

CALCIUM METABOLISM & HOMEOSTASIS

Calcium metabolism and its homeostasis mainly involves bone, kidney, gut, and parathyroid glands, depending on the activity of various hormones and pro-hormones, such as PTH, calcitonin, and vitamin D. Other factors (i.e. vitamins, medications, diet, and mobility) can also modify calcium metabolism. Serum calcium fractions are reported in (Fig. **2**).

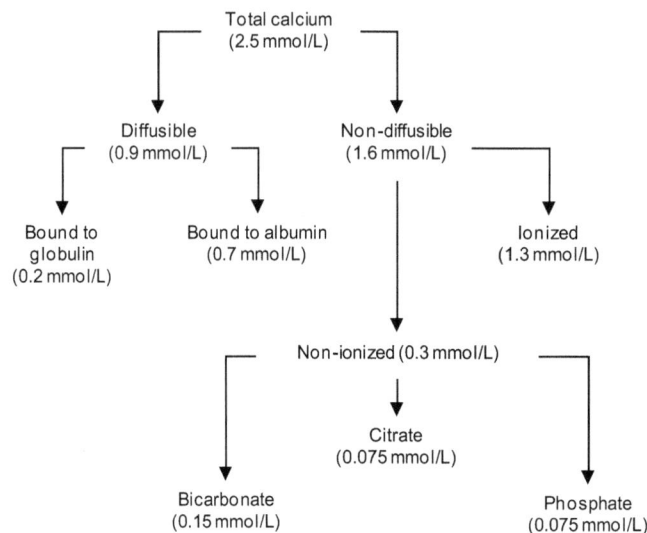

Figure 2: Serum calcium fractions.

A normal adult needs 500-1200 mg/day of calcium for the balancing of intake (diet and tissutal request) and losses (urine, stools, sweat). Dairy products (milk, cream, and cheese) are the principal sources of calcium intake. As mentioned above, calcium pool is divided in intracellular and extracellular. Intracellular calcium concentration should be very well defined according to its importance as a second (intracellular) messenger. The majority of extracellular calcium in the whole body is present in the form of hydroxylapatite (or hydroxyapatite) $[Ca_{10}(PO_4)_6(OH)_2]$, which represents the most important bone mineral. Up to 50% of bones are made up of a modified form of the inorganic mineral hydroxyapatite. The total normal extracellular calcium concentration (2.25 to 2.65 mmol/L, or 9 to 10.5 mg/dL) is divided into diffusible (bound to serum proteins like albumin or globulin) and non diffusible (distinct in ionized, or free calcium, and non ionized, calcium-complexes with phosphate, citrate and bicarbonate). Changes in pH levels can modify extracellular calcium levels: acidosis decreases albumin-bind calcium, while alcalosis decreases free calcium levels. Many other clinical conditions can increase or reduce extracellular pool of calcium.

PTH is a hormone synthesized and released by parathyroid glands as a straight-chain polypeptide, containing 84 amino acids. It checks the distribution of calcium and phosphate in the body. Secretion of PTH is strictly controlled by extracellular calcium levels through a negative feed-back, which is achieved by the activation of calcium-sensing receptors located on parathyroid cells. Calcium sensing receptors work by activating the phospholypase C pathway, through a guanylyl nucleotide binding protein (G protein), which increases intracellular calcium concentration. The sites of PTH actions are the bones, kidneys and gut (Table **1**).

Table 1: Parathyroid hormone actions. RANKL = receptor activator of nuclear actor-κ ligand.

Site	Effect
Bone	Enhances the release of calcium by an indirect stimulation of osteoclast mediated by osteoblast and RANK-RANKL system
Kidney	Enhances active reabsorption of calcium (and magnesium) from distal tubules and thick ascending limb
	Reduces reabsorption of phosphate from the proximal tubule
Intestine (via kidney)	Enhances absorption of calcium in the intestine by increasing the production of 1,25 dihydroxycholecalciferol [1,25(OH)$_2$D]

Its action is both direct (kidney) and indirect, mediated by vitamin D in the gut, and by osteoblasts and osteoclasts in the bone. In the presence of prolonged exposure to high serum levels of PTH, as occurs in patients with primary hyperparathyroidism, osteoclast activity predominates, leading to progressive bone resorption and hypercalcemia (see Chapter 2). PTH also increases the activity of the enzyme 1α-hydroxylase, which converts 25-hydroxycholecalciferol to 1, 25-dihydroxychole-calciferol [1, 25 (OH)$_2$D], the active form of vitamin D required for calcium uptake by intestinal cells, and reabsorption of calcium and phosphate by renal tubules.

Calcitonin is a hormone produced by C cells (parafollicular) in the thyroid gland that lowers the levels of calcium and phosphate in the blood. PTH action on extracellular calcium levels is opposed to the calcitonin action which primarily inhibits osteoclastic activity.

Vitamin D is a group of fat-soluble pro-hormones that enhances the absorption of calcium and phosphorus from the gut, and promotes their deposition in the bone (Table **2**).

Table 2: Vitamin D groups.

Vitamin D type	Characteristics
D_1	Molecular compound of ergacalciferol with lumisterol 1:1
D_2	Ergocalciferol, made from ergosterol, not produced by vertebrates
D_3	Cholecalciferol, made from 7-dehydrocholesterol in the skin
D_4	22-dihydroergocalciferol
D_5	Sitocalciferol, made from 7-dehydrocholesterol

Vitamin D_3 (cholecalciferol) is the endogenous form of vitamin D, but its synthesis is non-enzymatic. Vitamin D_3 is produced by the action of sunlight, when the UV (290-310 nm) light index is greater than

3, and from 7-dehydrocholesterol, a cholesterol metabolite widely distributed within the skin. No natural dietary source of this vitamin is currently available. Vitamin D_2 (ergocalciferol) is produced by UV irradiation of ergosterol, a plant sterol, and it usually represents a fortified tool for dairy products. Both vitamin D_2 and D_3 have the same metabolism and power (40 UI = 1 μg), but they are inactive. In the liver, vitamin D_3 is hydrossilated to $25(OH)D_3$, and then in the kidneys to $1,25(OH)_2D_3$ (calcitriol), where its production is favored by low serum calcium and phosphorus, and high PTH levels. The calcitriol actions are reported in Table **3**.

Table 3: Calcitriol actions.

Calcitriol actions
Stimulate osteoclastic resorption of calcium from bone
Facilitate the effect that PTH has on calcium resorption from bone
Increase kidney tubular absorption of calcium
Increase calcium absorption from gastrointestinal tract

Thus, calcitriol represents the active form of vitamin D_3 found in the body. It increases the flow of calcium into the bloodstream in several ways, and inhibits PTH secretion from the parathyroid gland (Fig. **3**). In addition, other paracrine and endocrine factors may influence calcium metabolism, including osteoclast activating factors, such as cytokines, interleukin-1 (IL-1), tumor necrosis factor (TNF), and transforming growth factor-beta (TGF-β). They are especially involved in the pathogenesis of malignancy-related hypercalcemia (see Chapter 3).

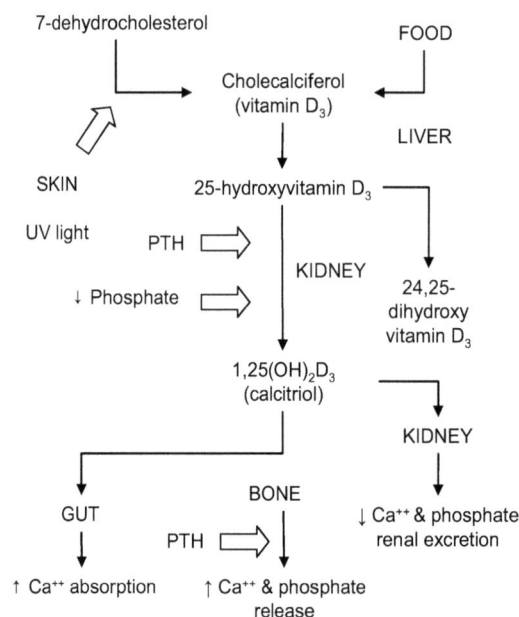

Figure 3: Pathways of vitamin D_3 activation.

Recent evidence showed that calcium metabolism is regulated by other factors such as fibroblast growth factor-23 (FGF-23) and Klotho, which are essential for maintaining calcium-phosphate homeostasis and regulating vitamin D metabolism as well as by the transient receptor potential cation channel, subfamily V, member 5 (TRPV5) [1].

The FGF-23 gene (located on chromosome 12) is a member of the fibroblast growth factor family (FGF) and encodes a protein corresponding to an old protein named phosphatonin [2], which is responsible for phosphate metabolism. The product of this gene inhibits renal tubular phosphate transport, increases urinary excretion of phosphorus, and inhibits renal production of 1,25$(OH)_2$D, thereby decreasing PTH serum levels and its production [3]. Mutations in FGF-23 gene lead to increased activity of FGF-23, and the renal phosphate loss found in autosomal dominant hypophosphatemic rickets [4]. FGF-23 is also overproduced by some types of tumors, causing tumor-produced osteomalacia [5]. Loss of FGF-23 activity leads to a phosphate level increase, and familial tumor calcinosis syndrome [6-7]. Higher levels of FGF-23 in patients with the end stage renal disease (ESRD), are independently correlated with a higher risk of mortality [8]. (Fig. **4**).

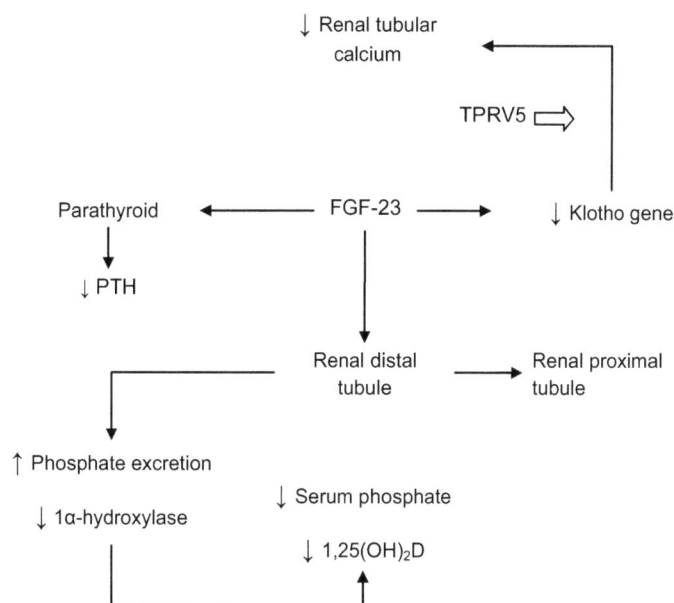

Figure 4: Actions of FGF-23, TPRV5, and Klotho gene on calcium metabolism.

TRPV5 is a human gene member of the transient receptor family and the TRP subfamily V. The calcium-selective channel TRPV5, encoded by this gene, has 6 transmembrane-spanning domains, multiple potential phosphorylation sites, a N-linked glycosylation site, and 5 ankyrin repeats (ANK). This protein forms homotetramers or heterotetramers, and is activated by a low internal calcium level that constitutes the apical Ca^{++} entry pathway in the process of active Ca^{++} reabsorption [9]. Klotho gene codes for a transmembrane protein that, in addition to other effects, provides some control over the sensitivity of the organism to insulin, and it appears to be involved in the aging process. Klotho gene deletion influences the spatial distribution of osteocytes and the synthesis of bone matrix proteins in addition to the accelerated aging of bone cells. Thus, not only reducing osteoblastic population but also disturbing bone mineralization [10-11]. Klotho-deficient mice manifest a syndrome resembling accelerated human aging and display extensive and accelerated arteriosclerosis. Additionally, they exhibit impaired endothelium dependent vasodilatation and impaired angiogenesis, suggesting that Klotho protein may protect the cardiovascular system through endothelium-derived NO production [12]. Klotho-deficient mice show increased production of vitamin D and altered mineral-ion homeostasis, which is suggested to be a cause of premature aging-like phenotypes. The lowering of vitamin D activity by dietary restriction reverses the premature aging-like phenotypes and prolongs survival in these mutants. These results suggest that aging-like phenotypes were due to Klotho-associated vitamin D metabolic abnormalities (hypervitaminosis) [13-14].

PATHOPHYSIOLOGY OF HYPERCALCEMIA

Usually, the kidney protects from hypercalcemia. Table **4** reports the sites of calcium reabsorption in the kidney.

Table 4: Sites of calcium reabsorption in the kidney.

Condition	Proximal tubule	TALH	Distal tubule
Hypercalcemia	↓	↓	↓
Hypocalcemia	↑	↑	Unknown
Hyperphosphatemia	Unknown	Unknown	↑
Hypophosphatemia	↓	Unknown	↓
Loud excess	↓	Unknown	↓
Acidosis	↓	Unknown	↓
Alcalosis	↑	Unknown	Unknown
PTH	↑	↑	↑
Calcitonin	Unknown	↑	↑
Insulin, glucose	↓	Unknown	↓

TALH = thick ascending limb of Henle's loop

However, in some cases hypercalciuria occurs before hypercalcemia, reducing the extracellular pool of calcium, while only in a few cases the kidney contributes to the development of hypercalcemia. An amount of calcium goes through the renal tubular cells according to an electrochemical gradient, but the complex cellular-membrane avoids penetration of high charged ions like calcium. The causes of hypercalcemia are reported in Table **5**.

Table 5: Causes of hypercalcemia. MEN = multiple endocrine neoplasia, PTHrP = parathyroid hormone-related protein, PTH = parathyroid hormone.

Common	Uncommon
HYPERPARATHYROIDISM	HEREDITARY DISEASES
Primary	MEN type I or II
Secondary	Familial hypocalciuric hypercalcemia
Tertiary in chronic renal failure	GRANULOMATOUS DISEASES
Posttransplantation	Sarcoidosis
Familial non MEN	DRUG INDUCED
MALIGNANCY	Lithium
Humoral hypercalcemia (PTHrP)	Vitamins A & D
Lytic bone disease (myeloma, leukemia)	Thiazides
Ectopic 1,25(OH)$_2$ vitamin D	Estrogens, androgens
Ectopic PTH (rare)	OTHERS
	Milk-alkali syndrome
	Immobilization
	Recovery from renal failure
	Rhabdomyolysis

Calcium channels and carriers are the best way through which the calcium enters into renal tubular cells. They should be divided into L-type calcium channels and other specific calcium channels, and are identified in the S2 region of proximal tubules, in the cortical thick ascending limb of Henle's loop

(TALH), in distal convoluted tubules and in cortical collecting ducts. The quantity of calcium filtrated by the glomeruli is the result of the GFR, and ultra filtrate calcium (UFCa). Considering a healthy adult with 100 mL/min of GFR and 54 mg/L of UFCa, calcium filtrated from glomeruli is about 8 g/day. Renal tubules have to absorb again 98-99% of calcium filtrated by the glomeruli to keep a neutral daily calcium balance. Obligatory losses, 150-200 mg/day are balanced with intestinal absorption of calcium mediated by vitamin D in the presence of PTH.

The threshold of renal calcium sensibility in healthy adults, is set at 9 mg/dL at an extracellular level, but the threshold may change. In hypoparathyroidism the threshold decreases from 9 mg/dL to 6.5 mg/dl whereas in hyperthyroidism it increases from 9 mg/dL to 12 mg/dL. Renal calcium absorption depends on the gradient (proximal tubule) as well as the concentration of calcium levels (cortical TALH and distal tubule), as sodium does. Renal calcium excretion, more often, is similar to the renal sodium excretion. Both increase or decrease at the same time, and the consequence is that a low sodium diet intake in patients with hypercalciuria has turned out to be effective. Seventy percent of all the filtrated calcium by glomeruli, is reabsorbed by proximal tubule, 20% by TALH, from 5 to 10% by distal tubule, and less than 5% by cortical collecting ducts. Less than 3% of calcium filtrated by glomeruli appears in excreted urine. Without the presence of a PTH increase, there are two opposed effects on factors regulating calcium filtration. The first relates to a decrease in the filtration coefficient (Kf) causing a GFR decrement, while the second relates to an increase in the UFCa and in the levels of filtrated calcium. Both may lead to an overall increase in the renal calcium excretion. (Fig. **5**) shows the hormonal effects of hypercalcemia.

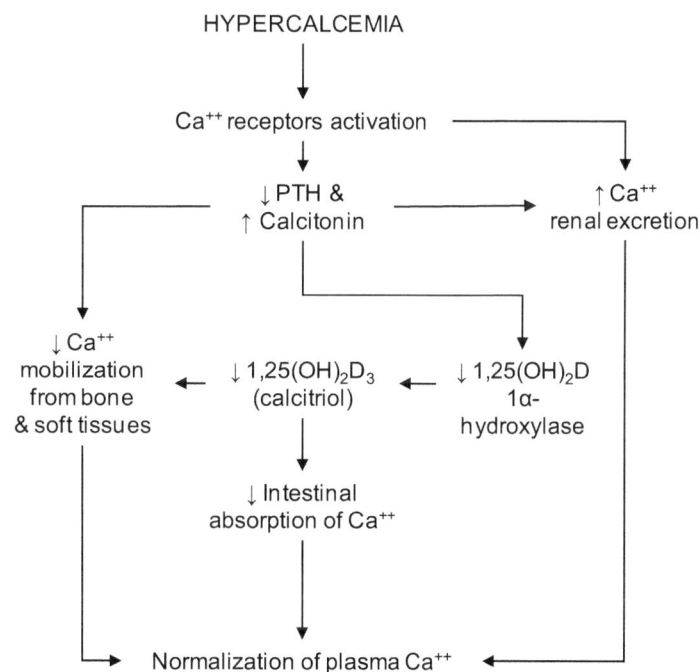

HYPERCALCEMIA
↓
Ca⁺⁺ receptors activation
↓
↓ PTH & ↑ Calcitonin → ↑ Ca⁺⁺ renal excretion

↓ Ca⁺⁺ mobilization from bone & soft tissues ← ↓ 1,25(OH)₂D₃ (calcitriol) ← ↓ 1,25(OH)₂D 1α-hydroxylase

↓ Intestinal absorption of Ca⁺⁺

Normalization of plasma Ca⁺⁺

Figure 5: Hormonal effects of hypercalcemia.

In the *vasa recta* and in chink, hypercalcemia induces an inhibition of the potassium channel because it stops the flow of potassium necessary to make the Na+/K+/2Cl- cotrasporter pump work correctly. Reduced activity of this carrier leads to a lower calcium, sodium and magnesium reabsorption in TALH. Oral loaded phosphate intake causes a decrease in the calcium excretion also by an extravascular volume increase. This effect is delayed and could be due to an increase in the secretion of the PTH which follows the free calcium decrease. An increased extravascular volume with isotonic saline solution causes an increase in the renal calcium and sodium excretion.

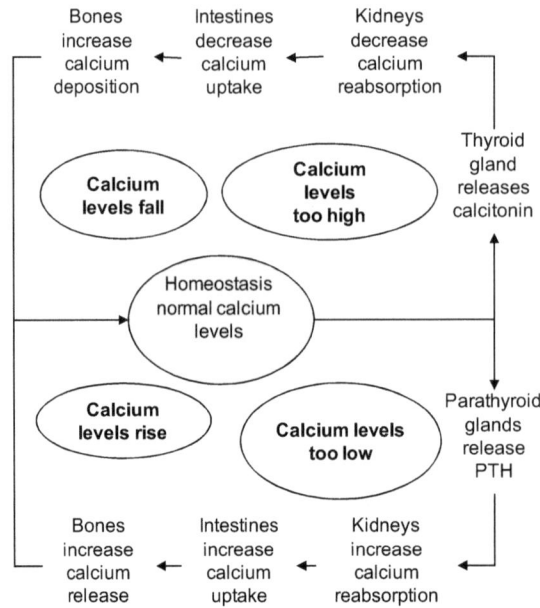

Figure 6: Mechanisms maintaining calcium homeostasis.

Acute and chronic metabolic acidosis are related to an increased calcium excretion in spite of the calcium filtrated modifications of PTH levels, whereas metabolic alkalosis decreases renal calcium loss. Respiratory pH alterations should cause the same modification as the metabolic pH alterations seen above, but no certain result has yet been found. Finally, insulin, glucagon and glucose, if given intravenously, may cause hypercalciuria. The chronic administration of mineralcorticoids (i.e. fluorohydrocortisone) causes massive sodium retention as well as enhanced calcium excretion, while diuretics can both increase (osmotic and loop diuretics) or reduce (thiazides, amiloride, spironolactone) renal calcium excretion. The mechanisms maintaining calcium homeostasis are shown in (Fig. **6**).

NEPHROLITHIASIS & NEPHROCALCINOSIS

Nephrolithiasis is defined as the condition of stones-forming inside the renal tubules or inside the collecting duct, but stones can be often localized in the urinary duct or inside the bladder. Nephrolithiasis, also defined as urolithiasis, has been noted to occur in the setting of therapeutic drug use, with crystals of drug forming within the renal tract in some patients currently treated with indinavir or triamterene. The various types of stones and their frequency are shown in (Fig **7**).

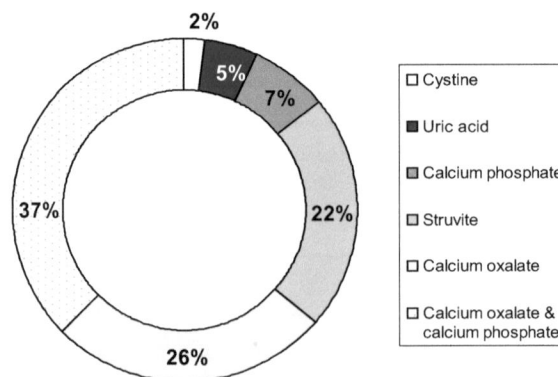

Figure 7: Type of stones in nephrolithiasis.

The clinical features of nephrolithiasis can be different, depending on the type, size and abode of the stone (Table **6**). Small kidney stones can leave the body, passing in urine stream without symptoms, and 90 % of stones of 4 mm or less in size usually will pass spontaneously. If stones grow to sufficient size before passage, they can cause an obstruction of the ureter, with subsequent dilatation or stretching of the upper ureter and renal pelvis, causing ureteral muscle spasms.

Table 6: Clinical presentation of nephrolithiasis.

Presentation	Features
Pain (ureteral colic, loin pain, dysuria)	Revolves with stone passage or removal May migrate anteriorly or inferiorly Nausea, vomiting, frequency, hematuria may be present
Hematuria	May be microscopic or macroscopic depends on large calculi Differential diagnosis: tumor, infection, glomerular renal disease
Urinary tract infection	May be recurrent, chronic or acute
Asymptomatic urine abnormality	Microscopic hematuria Proteinuria Batteriuria
Acute renal failure (if bilateral renal tract obstruction or unilateral in single functioning kidney)	Interruption of urinary flow

As a consequence patients feel pain, most commonly localized in the flank, lower abdomen, and groin. This, named renal colic, is the most typical clinical feature of nephrolithiasis, and is usually observed in association with hematuria, due to a damage of the lining of the urinary tract, which may be either macroscopic or microscopic. Nausea and vomiting, frequently, occur as well. About 99% of stones larger than 6 mm require some form of intervention. Epidemiologic traits of nephrolithiasis are shown in Table **7**.

Table 7: Epidemiology of nephrolithiasis.

Parameter	Characteristics
Gender	Male: Female from 2:1 to 4:1
Annual incidence	1:1000
Prevalence	Increased in the last decades (3.2% in the '70s; 5.2% in the '90s) Increased with age until 70 in men and 60 in women
Incidence peaks	Third and fourth decades
Race	Caucasians are most likely
Geographic distribution	Depends on sunlight exposure (increased sweating and urine concentration, enhanced vitamin D production)

The pathogenesis of stone forming is a result of an alteration in the balancing of the urinary tissue between a sovrasaturation of ions usually present and a decreased concentration of substances (i.e. citrate and thiosulfate) that normally prevent ion precipitation [15, 16].

This process can be a result of impaired cellular function due to intrinsic mechanism or triggered by external stimuli which in turn calls for an optimal range of urinary pH to work at its best [17]. Each condition able to modify this balance can be responsible for stone forming that, in the long run, can induce chronic kidney disease (CKD) [18]. The pathogenesis of nephrolithiasis is shown in (Fig. **8**).

ALTERED BALANCE

Increased ionic constituents ←→ Decrease ionic constituents
(i.e. citrate)

Sovrasaturation

pH ⟹ ↓

Nucleation

↓

Aggregation

↓

Anchoring

↓

Renal Stone

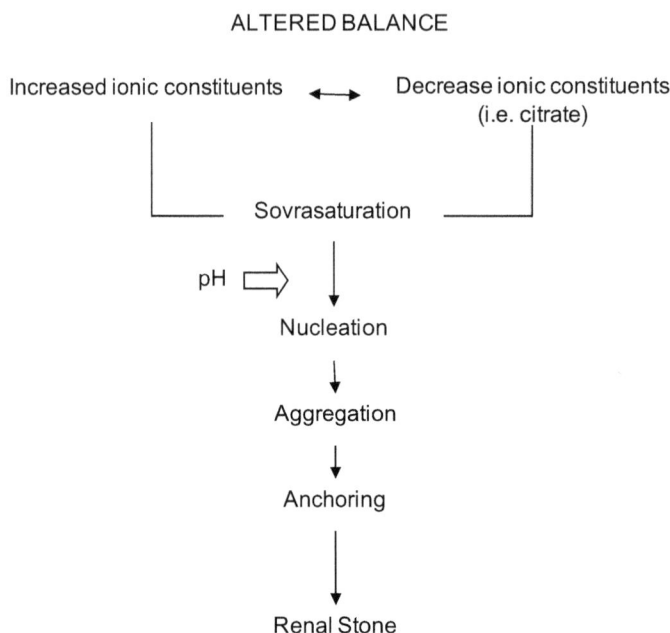

Figure 8: Pathogenesis of nephrolythyasis.

Underlying abnormality of the kidney, infections of the urinary tract, and dehydration can support development of renal stones. All patients having a single kidney stone in their clinical history should undergo a basic evaluation, while the others should undergo further clinical and biochemical investigations (Table **8**). A correct approach to the diagnosis takes into consideration familial and clinical history, physical examination, laboratory findings, and radiological tests. When possible, a chemical analysis of the stone(s) should also be obtained.

Table 8: Patients need basic and complete investigations. PTH = parathyroid hormone, CT = computed tomography scanning.

Patients need basic investigation	Patients need a complete investigation
Medical and family history	Patients with metabolically active stones (stones increasing in number and size in 1 year)
Medications	Children
Lifestyle, occupation	Non calcium stone formers
Diet, fluid intake	Non caucasian
Physical examination	
Laboratory data: urinalysis, urine culture, stone analysis	
Blood chemistry: renal function, calcium (if elevated PTH) sodium, potassium, chloride, bicarbonate, uric acid, phosphorus	
Imaging: plain abdominal X-ray, ultrasonography intravenous urography, abdominal CT	

The first step of treatment is pain relief using non steroidal anti-inflammatory drugs, such as kerotolac (previously intramuscularly or intravenously, and then orally) or opiates, giving general suggestions (Table **9**).

Table 9: General treatment of nephrolithiasis.

General treatment
Fluid intake (greater than 2-2.5 liters daily especially in the evening because during the night the urine concentration is physiologically increased)
Salt intake (2 g/day; sodium increased calcium excrection)
Reduce animal protein intake (several mechanism such as generation of sulfate ions; increased calcium release from bones, decreased renal tubule calcium reabsorption, decreased urinary citrate excretion due to metabolic acidosis
Normal calcium intake in order to age and gender

The second step is performing general and specific strategies to prevent stone formation, as reported in Table **10**. In case of failure of medical treatment, patients should undergo surgical therapies, including endoscopic o percutaneus techniques, such as cystoscopic placement of ureteral stent, extracorporeal shock wave lithotripsy, or nephrostomy with urine drainage (Table **11**).

Nephrocalcinosis, once known as Albright's calcinosis, means a presence of elevated calcium content within the kidney. Originally, this term was used to describe deposition of calcium salts in the renal parenchyma due to primary hyperparathyroidism (HPT), while it is now commonly used to describe diffuse and fine renal parenchymal calcifications. This situation can be symmetric but, in case of anatomic disorders such as medullary sponge kidney, it can be unilateral. There is no correlation between extension of calcifications and renal impairment. According to the sites of calcifications, nephrocalcinosis can be divided into medullary nephrocalcinosis (MN) and cortical nephrocalcinosis (CN).

Table 10: Specific treatments of stone disease.

Condition	Treatment
Hypercalciuria	Thiazide diuretic (chlorthalidone or indapamide; check potassium level)
Enteric Hyperoxaluria	Diet Calcium carbonate, potassium citrate Magnesium
Primary Hyperoxaluria	Pyridoxine (in Type 1) Potassium and magnesium supplementation Ortophosphate (with creatinine clearance > 50 mL/min) Liver and renal transplantation
Hypocitraturia	Potassium citrate
Hyperuricosuria	Low-purine diet Allopurinol
Uric acid stones	Potassium citrate Acetazolamide Low-purine diet Low-animal protein diet Allopurinol
Struvite stones (infection stones or triple-phosphate stones)	Culture-specific antibiotic Acetohydroxamic acid (?) Chemolysis (?) Surgical techniques
Cystine stones	Increasing urine volume (4 litres) Low sodium diet D-penicillamine Captopril

Any disorder leading to hypercalcemia or hypercalciuria may cause MN, and in this case, parenchimal calcifications are usually bilateral and symmetric. In primary hyperoxaluria or in hyperoxaluria following bariatric surgery, calcifications can deposit in both medullary and cortical site [19].

Table 11: Surgical indications of stone diseases.

Urosepsis	Hematuria requiring transfusion
Intractable pain	Staghorn calculi
Bilateral disease involving acute renal failure or monolateral disease in single kidney)	Stone growth despite optima medical treatment
Persistent obstruction	Size of calculi > 7 mm

The common causes for MN vary according to age, as well as many hereditary disorders are associated with MN (Table **12**). In X-linked hypercalciuric nephrolithiasis, mutations affecting the voltage-gated chloride ion channel-5 (CLCN5) gene on the X-chromosome lead to inactivation of CLC-5. Clinical features include hypofosfatemia, hypercalciuria, nephrolithiasis, nephrocalcinosis, aminoaciduria, hematuria, proteinuria, glycosuria, renal failure, and rickets.

Table 12: Causes of medullary nephrocalcinosis

Non-hereditary	Hereditary
Each cause of hypercalcemia	X-linked hypercalciuric nephrolithiasis (dent disease)
Medullary sponge kidney	Primary hypomagnesemia-hypercalciuria
Renal tubular acidosis (specifically distal RTA)	Bartter's syndrome
Renal tuberculosis	
Renal papillary necrosis	
Hyperoxaluria	

Primary hypomagnesemia-hypercalciuria syndrome is a rare autosomal recessive condition, in which a defective production of paracellin-1, a protein of the cellular tight-junction occurs. This protein is necessary for calcium and magnesium reabsorption in TALH. Clinical features include urinary tract infections, polyuria, seizures, hypercalciuria, hypermagnesuria, urinary-concentrating defect, renal failure and ESRD, requiring renal replacement therapy. Hearing disorders and ocular impairment may also be observed. In Bartter's syndrome several autosomal recessive genetic mutations are possible, leading to clinical features similar to excessive loop-diuretic intake, such as hypercalciuria, nephrocalcinosis, and nephrolithiasis. Cortical nephrocalcinosis is the result of parenchimal tissue destruction secondary to infarction, infection or tumors. It is usually asymmetric and localized in the renal cortex. Causes of CN include renal transplant rejection, tuberculosis, cortical necrosis, and chronic glomerulonephritis (Table **13**).

Table 13: Causes of cortical nephrocalcinosis.

Acute cortical necrosis	Renal transplant rejection
Chronic glomerulonephritis	Sickle cell disease (rare)
Alport syndrome	Vitamin B6 deficiency (rare)
Prolonged hypercalcemia/hypercalciuria	

The treatment of nephrolithiasis and nephrocalcinosis is similar. It consists of removing the underlying disease and reducing hypercalcemia, hyperphosfatemia and oxalosis in order to prevent further calcium deposits.

NEPHROPATHY, RENAL FAILURE & HYPERCALCEMIA

Hypercalcemia impairs the urinary concentrating ability, leading to different renal alterations, such as disturbance of tubular function, nephrolithiasis, and renal failure. The main causes of hypercalcemia are reported in Table **5**.

Hypercalcemia is likely to occur in patients with acute renal failure and it is usually seen in the recovery from rhabdomyolysis. In this situation, calcium can be set free from calcium-containing complexes inside muscles. In addition, secondarily to the increased calcitriol production from a recovered kidney, a larger effect due to the PTH action is observed. In these situations, calcium levels are not usually dangerous, and they can be cut down by loop diuretics or temporary dialysis treatment.

Hypercalcemia can also occurs in the elderly with gradual a softening of the bones, and in patients fed for a long time with total parenteral nutrition (TPN). It can give origin to a vicious cycle, making perpetual the hypercalcemia until a large calcium intake appears. Kidney involvement can be reversible stopping calcium intake, but in the long run it can lead to the ESRD. Kidney alterations are localized in the distal straight and convoluted tubule, and in the collecting duct. They are caused by an obstruction due to calcium salts or epithelial custs, or by the hemodynamic alteration (vasoconstriction) as a consequence of a direct effect of calcium on vascular tone, that leads to a reduction of renal blood flow and GFR. Hypercalcemia and increased PTH levels, if present, further decrease both Kf and GFR. The clinical features are reported in Table **14**. Nephrogenic diabetes insipidus due to a partial insensibility to antidiuretic hormone (ADH) causes polyuria (at least 2.5 litres over 24 hours in adults), and subsequently polydipsia.

The aim of the treatment is to get rid of the causes of hypercalcemia, but if calcium levels are above 3.5 mmol/L, an adequate therapy should be started.

Table 14: Signs & symptoms of patients with nepholithiasis and hypercalcemia.

Symptoms due to nephrolithiasis	Symptoms due to hypercalcemia
Loin pain	Gastro-intestinal: anorexia, nausea, vomiting pancreatitis (uncommon)
Microhematuria, macrohematuria	Muscle weakness, asthenia
Renal colic	Neurological: depression, lethargy
	Renal: polyuria, renal failure, nephrolithiasis, nephrocalcinosis
	Cardiac: QT tract alterations, arrhythmia, cardiac stroke
	Polydipsia
	Dehydration

Rehydration helps decrease calcium level through dilution, eliminating excess calcium through the urine. The rate of rehydration is based upon the severity of hypercalcemia and dehydration, as well as the ability of the patient to tolerate rehydration.

For mild-to-moderate elevations of calcium, patients are usually directed to increase oral fluid intake. When the water pool is set up again, loop diuretics, able to increase renal calcium loss and blocking renal calcium reabsorption, should be used. Calcitonin has a transient effect, whereas bisphosphonates usually represent the drug of choice (see Chapter 8). In non-responders to pharmacological treatment, hemodialysis treatment without calcium is required. This strategy should be the first choice in patient already undergoing a renal replacement therapy.

RENAL TRANSPLANTATION & HYPERCALCEMIA

Progress of secondary HPT after renal transplantation and its prevention and resolution have not yet been defined. When ESRD occurs, secondary HPT causes important skeletal abnormalities. This bone disease has a wide spectrum of alterations, mainly depending on severity and duration of ESRD, characteristics of dialysis, and calcitriol and PTH levels. It can be divided into three different types, according to the cellular turn-over.

Normal turn-over pattern (light osteopathy) is characterized by a slight increase of the bone remodeling processes, and its frequency varies from 15% to 30%

High turn-over pattern (*osteitis fibrosa cystica*, von Recklinghausen's disease of bone) is a skeletal disorder occurring in patients with long-standing secondary HPT, with a subsequent increase in the number of both osteoblasts and osteoclasts. Thus, bone resorption increases, and minerals, including calcium, go through the bone into the bloodstream. In addition, an over-activity of this process results in a loss of the bone mass and weakening of bones, as their calcified supporting structures are replaced by fibrous tissue (peritrabecular fibrosis), with cyst-like brown tumors formation in and around the bone. The frequency of high turned-over pattern varies from 50% to 70% of patients with ESRD.

Low turn-over pattern includes osteomalacia and adynamic bone disease. Many of the effects of osteomalacia overlap with the more common osteoporosis, but the two diseases are significantly different. Osteomalacia is characterized by an incomplete mineralization of the bone protein framework, known as osteoid. Some years ago, osteomalacia was thought to be correlated to the aluminum hydroxide (used as antiacid and calcium binding) accumulation, but the aluminum-associated bone disease (AABD) is now uncommon. Its frequency is decreasing from 20-40% in the early 80's to 4-6% nowadays. Most ESDR patients with osteomalacia show a clear deficiency of vitamin D, a mineral deficiency or both.

The second disorder is characterized by a lack of the remodeling processes and the presence of a very small number of osteoblasts on bone biopsy. PTH levels are very low (real deficit, or functional deficit related to a skeletal resistance). In patients with adynamic bone disease (ABD) episodes, hypercalcemia occurs more often than in those with high turn-over skeletal lesions. The frequency of ABD is unclear, ranging between 15% and 50%, but it seems to be more frequent in diabetic patients and in those with ESRD in peritoneal dialysis. Renal transplantation corrects the majority of pathogenetic conditions leading to secondary HPT, such as diminished renal calcitriol production, skeletal resistance to the calcemic action of PTH and hyperphosphatemia (Table **15**).

Table 15: Pathogenesis of secondary hyperparathyroidism.

Hypocalcemia	Modification of regulation of pre-pro-PTH gene transcription
Reduced renal calcitriol production	Reduced expression of receptors for vitamin D and calcium in parathyroid glands
Skeletal resistance to the calcemic action of PTH	Hyperphosphatemia following reduced renal phosphate excretion

However, increasing levels of PTH have been observed for many years in 50% of patients who underwent renal transplantation, while only 5-10% may have a normal bone not longer than 1-2 years from renal graft. In this setting, pre-transplantation serum PTH is the marker of choice, but factors like age, duration of renal replacement therapy and renal function of kidney donors, should also be considered, as well as genetic factors, such as homozygosis for deletion of restriction enzymes Bsm I and ApA I [20-22].

Pretransplantation parathyroid glands function represents an important predictor of posttransplantation calcium levels, that are higher in patients with high PTH levels than in those with normal PTH [23]. This is due to a higher sensibility of target cells to PTH following a reduction of resistance, due to the uremic state or following an increase of intestinal absorption. PTH presents an altered secretive kinetics, and its production from parathyroid glands is not correlated to extracellular calcium levels. Reduced density of calcitriol receptors and decreased expression of calcium membrane receptors make the cells more resistant to physiologic concentration of calcitriol and calcium. In case of parathyroidectomy, anatomic response is, more often, nodular hyperplasia that we know to be connected with lower expression of calcium-receptor. High pretransplantation serum PTH levels protect against hypocalcemia within the first postoperative week, but put patients at risk for hypercalcemia later [23]. Resolution of soft-tissue calcifications, high dose of corticosteroids therapy after transplantation, and immobilization are factors that contribute to the development of hypercalcemia.

Three different types of clinical consequences of persisting secondary HPT should be considered: (1) bone disease (renal osteodistrophy, osteopenic-osteoporotic syndrome, aseptic osteonecrosis, and pathological fractures), (2) non-bone diseases, and (3) graft diseases. Non-bone consequences are acute pancreatitis that occurs in 3% of patients, but can lead to mortality in 70% of those affected by cardiovascular impairment [24]. In renal graft, clinical consequences are due to an acute tubulonecrosis following elevated PTH levels. This finding is described in 40% of patients undergoing renal transplantation and it can lead to a worsened function of renal graft [25]. Calcium channel blockers seem to be able to prevent this clinical feature [26] (see Chapter 8).

Laboratory findings include hypophosphoremia, and mild to moderate hypercalcemia, with high PTH levels. Hypophosporemia, independent of PTH levels, is observed in almost 40% of patients. It may represent either an alteration of renal tubular function or a pharmacological interference (i.e. steroids). In patients with optimal renal graft function, hypophosphoremia may increase hypercalcemia after stimulating the 1 α-hydroxilase in renal proximal tubule.

The objective of the treatment is to achieve PTH levels within range, according to guideline suggestions of pre- and posttransplantation. The calcium-sensing receptor antagonists (the use of which is forbidden for the time being in post-transplant hyper-PTH) unless used in off-label condition, correct hypercalcemia and PTH by increasing urinary calcium excretion, simultaneously improving BMD [27-28]. They can reduce bone and muscle problems of the patients, and the worsening of their quality of life, the improvement of which is one of the targets of renal transplantation [28-29]. Dual-energy x-ray absorptiometry is the technique of choice for monitoring BMD and measuring bone density at the spine and hip [30] (see Chapter 6).

Oral calcium and vitamin D supplements are effective for patients with reduced BMD, while bisphosphonates, which inhibit the osteoclast activity, are effective in the treatment of post-transplant osteopenia (see Chapter 8). Bisphosphonates, as well as calcitriol, reduce bone loss and increase bone mass but, unfortunately, their effectiveness on fracture rate is still unclear. Surgical treatment (see Chapter 7) must be taken into consideration, not later than 6 months from transplantation, if medical management is ineffective [31] (Table **16**).

Table 16: Surgical indications.

Tertiary hyperparathyroidism (severe hypercalcemia for more than 6-12 months	Calcium-related renal allograft dysfunction
Symptomatic or progressive hypercalcemia	Progressive vascular calcifications
Nephrolithiasis	Calciphylaxis
Persistent metabolic bone disease	

CONCLUSIONS

Calcium is an ion necessary for the human body and its metabolism. For this reason calcium level must be kept steady, since hypercalcemia can lead to different organ impairment. The relationship between hypercalcemia and kidney has been analyzed, but problems related to the cardiovascular (i.e. arrhythmia, arterial hypertension) and neuromuscular system (clinical feature simulating an amyotrophic lateral sclerosis), as well as those related to the skin (calciphylaxis) should be considered. Calciphylaxis is a rare but potentially dangerous form of skin necrosis, which can lead to death in 60-80% of cases, due to sepsis from necrotic skin lesions [31, 32].

Basic mechanism regulating calcium metabolism have long been defined, but the complete role of new factors, such as FGF-23, TRPV5, and Klotho gene, is still under study. Advances in the understanding of their mechanisms of action will be crucial, having several practical consequences in the treatment and prevention of hypercalcemya. This would allow to move from a support therapy, sometimes ineffective, to a specific and addressed therapy, especially in patients with chronic hypercalcemic conditions.

The administration of new classes of drugs, such as calcium-sensing receptor antagonists, regulating calcium-sensing receptors, has shown to be effective especially in patients under renal replacement therapy and secondary HPT. They powerfully reduce PTH and calcium serum levels in more than 50% of such a patients, but the use of these drugs in patients with renal failure not yet under dialysis treatment, as well as in those with HPT persisting after renal transplantation, is still under consideration. The reduction of the incidence of renal ostheodistrophy may lead both to a significant improvement of quality of life in all nephropatic patients, either under renal replacement therapy or posttransplantation therapy, and to a reduction of cardiovascular events (i.e. early heart and vascular calcifications)

REFERENCES

[1]   Medici D, Razzaque MS, DeLuca S, *et al*. FGF-23-Klotho signaling stimulates proliferation and prevents vitamin D-induced apoptosis. J Cell Biol 2008; 182: 459-465.

[2]   Strewler GJ: FGF23, hypophosphatemia and rickets: has phosphorylation been found ? Proc Natl Acad Sci 2001; 98: 5945-5946.

[3]   Fukagawa M, Kazama JJ. With or without the kidney: the role of FGF 23 in CKD. Nephrol Dial Transplant 2005; 20: 1295-1298.

[4]   Shimada T, Muto T, Urakawa I, *et al*. Mutant FGF-23 responsible for autosomal dominant hypophosphatemic rickets in resistant to proteolithic cleavage and causes hypophosphatemia in vivo. Endocrinology 2002; 143: 3179-3182.

[5]   White KE, Jonsson KB, Carn G, *et al*. The autosomal dominant hypophosphatemic rickets (ADHR) gene is a secreted polypeptide overexpressed by tumors that cause phosphate wasting. J Clin Endocrinol Metab 2001; 86: 497-500.

[6]   Benet-Pages A, Orlik P, Strom MT, Lorenz-Depiereux B. An FGF 23 missense mutation causes familial tumoral calcinosis with hyperphosphatemia. Hum Mol Genet 2005; 14: 385-390.

[7]   Chefetz I, Heller R, Galli-Tsinopoulou A, *et al*. A novel homozygous missense mutation in FGF 23 causes tumoral calcinosis associated with disseminated visceral calcification. Hum Genet 2005; 118: 261-266.

[8]   Gutierrez OM, Mannstadt M, Isakova T, *et al*. Fibroblast growth factor 23 and mortality among patients undergoing hemodialisys. N Engl J Med 2008; 359: 584-592.

[9]   Gkika D, Mahieu F, Nilius B, Hoenderop JG, Bindels RJ. 80K-H as a new Ca2+ sensor regulating the activity of the epithelial Ca2+ channel transient receptor potential cation channel V5 (TRPV5). J Biol Chem 2004; 279: 26351-26357.

[10] Suzuki H, Amizuka N, Oda K, Noda M, Ohshima H, Maeda T. Histological and elemental analyses of impaired bone mineralization in klotho-deficient mice. J Anat 2008; 212: 275-285.

[11] Suzuki H, Amizuka N, Oda K, *et al*. Histological evidence of the altered distribution of osteocytes and bone matrix synthesis in klotho-deficient mice. Arch Histol Cytol 2005; 68: 371-381.

[12] Kurosu H, Yamamoto M, Clark JD, *et al*. Suppression of aging in mice by the hormone Klotho. Science 2005; 309: 1829-1833.

[13] Tsujikawa H, Kurotaki Y, Fujimori T, Fukuda K, Nabeshima Y. Klotho, a gene related to a syndrome resembling human premature aging, functions in a negative regulatory circuit of vitamin D endocrine system. Mol Endocrinol 2003; 17: 2393-2403.

[14] Imura A, Tsuji Y, Murata M, *et al*. Alpha-Klotho as a regulator of calcium homeostasis. Science 2007; 316 (5831): 1615-1618.

[15] Khan SR, Canales BK. Genetic basis of renal cellular dysfunction and the formation of kidney stones. Urol Res 2009; 37: 169-180.

[16] Asplin JR, Donahue SE, Lindeman C, *et al*. Thiosulfate reduces calcium phosphate nephrolithiasis. J Am Soc Nephrol 2009; 20: 1246-1253.

[17] Renkema KY, Velic A, Dijkman HB, *et al*. The calcium-sensing receptor promotes urinary acidification to prevent nephrolithiasis. J Am Soc Nephrol 2009; 20: 1705-1713.

[18] Rule AD, Bergstralh EJ, Melton LJ 3rd, *et al*. Kidney stones and the risk for chronic kidney disease. Clin J Am Soc Nephrol 2009; 4: 804-811.

[19] Whitson JM, Stackhouse GB, Stoller ML. Hyperoxaluria after modern bariatric surgery: case series and literature review. Int Urol Nephrol 2009. DOI 10.1007/s11255-009-9602-5.

[20] Messa P, Sindici C, Cannella G, *et al*. Persistent secondary hyperparathyroidism after renal transplantation. Kidney Int 1998; 54: 1704-1713.

[21] Fernandez E, Fibla A, Betrin A, *et al*. Association between vitamin D receptor polymorphism and relative hypoparathyroidism in patients with chronic renal failure. J Am Soc Nephrol 1997; 8: 1546-1552.

[22] Yokoyama K, Shigematsu T, Tsukada T, *et al*. ApA I polymorphism in the vitamin D receptor gene may affect the parathyroid response in Japanese with end-stage renal disease. Kidney Int 1998; 53: 454-458.

[23] Evenepoel P, Van den Bergh B, Naesens M, *et al*. Calcium metabolism in the early posttransplantation period. Clin J Am Soc Nephrol 2009; 4: 665-672.

[24] Fernandez JA, Rosemberg JC. Post-transplantation pancreatitis. Surg Gynecol Obstet 1976; 143: 795-798.

[25] Hall BM, Tiller DJ, Duggin GG, *et al*. Post-transplant acute renal failure in cadaver renal recipients treated with cyclosporine. Kidney Int 1985; 28: 178-186.

[26] Serra AL, Wuhrmann C, Wuthrich RP. Phosphatemic effect of cinacalcet in kidney transplant recipients with persistent Hypeparathyroidism. Am J Kidney Dis 2008; 52: 1151-1157.

[27] Borchhardt KA, Heinzl H, Mayerwoger E, *et al*. Cinacalcet increases calcium excretion in hypercalcemic hyperparathyroidism after kidney transplantation. Transplantation 2008; 86: 919-924.

[28] Bergua C, Torregrosa JV, Fuster D, *et al*. Effect of cinacalcet on hypercalcemia and bone mineral density in renal transplanted patients with secondary hyperparathyroidism. Transplantation 2008; 15: 413-417.

[29] Triponez F, Clark OH, Vanrenthergem Y, *et al*. Surgical treatment of persistent hyperparathyroidism after renal transplantation. Ann Surg 2008; 248: 18-30.

[30] Lumachi F, Camozzi V, Ermani, Nardi A, Luisetto G. Lumbar spine bone mineral density changes in patients with primary hyperparathyroidism according to age and gender. Ann N Y Acad Sci 2008; 1117: 362-366.

[31] Beitz JM. Calciphylaxis: an uncommon but potentially deadly form of skin necrosis. Am J Nurs 2004; 104: 36-37.

[32] Hitti WA, Papadimitriou JC, Bartlett S, *et al*. Spontaneous cutaneous ulcers in a patient with a moderate degree of chronic kidney disease: a different spectrum of calciphylaxis. Scand J Urol Nephrol 2008; 42: 181-183.

CHAPTER 2

Primary Hyperparathyroidism & Benign Diseases

Franco Lumachi[1] & Stefano M.M. Basso[2]

[1]*University of Padua, School of Medicine, 35128 Padova, Italy and* [2]*Division of Surgery I, S. Maria degli Angeli Hospital, 33170 Pordenone, Italy*

Abstract: Primary hyperparathyroidism (HPT) is the most common cause of hypercalcemia in non-hospitalized patients. Benign sporadic primary HPT is caused by a solitary adenoma in 80-85%, by multiglandular disease (multiple adenoma, parathyroid hyperplasia) in 12-14%, and parathyroid carcinoma in 1-2% of the cases. Parathyroid carcinoma is an uncommon finding, and its etiology remains unclear. Primary HPT can also occur in familial syndromes, such as multiple endocrine neoplasia type 1 (MEN 1), MEN 2A, hyperparathyroidism-jaw tumor (HPT-JT) syndrome, and familial isolated primary HPT, which seems to be an early stage of MEN 1 or HPT-JT. Most of the patients with primary HPT are diagnosed because of asymptomatic hypercalcemia, and both signs and symptoms of the disease, when present, are nonspecific, mainly depending on serum calcium concentration. Some patients, however, are diagnosed because of having osteopenia, osteoporosis, or unjustified recurrent bilateral nephrolithiasis. Primary HPT can be discovered by a simultaneous increase of both serum calcium and parathyroid hormone (PTH) levels, and thus the diagnosis can be obtained by inclusion rather than by excluding all the other causes of hypercalcemia. Indeed, the PTH measurement represents the keystone for differential diagnosis between primary HPT and malignancy-associated hypercalcemia. Other benign causes of hypercalcemia are drug-induced (vitamins A & D intoxication, thiazides, lithium, estrogens), endocrine (thyrotoxicosis), post-transplant and tertiary HPT, and familial benign hypocalciuric hypercalcemia. Virtually, all symptomatic patients with confirmed primary HPT should be referred for surgery, while more restrictive criteria have been suggested for the management of those with asymptomatic HPT.

INTRODUCTION

Primary hyperparathyroidism (HPT) is the most common cause of hypercalcemia in non-hospitalized patients, occurring in an estimated 0.2% to 0.5% of the population [1]. Calcium metabolism is mainly regulated by parathyroid glands, kidney, gut, and bone, depending on the activity of parathyroid hormone (PTH), vitamin D, and calcitonin, but other factors, such as fibroblast growth factor-23 (FGF-23) and Klotho, are necessary for maintaining calcium-phosphate homeostasis (see Chapter 1). Table **1** reports the old and new actors of calcium homeostasis.

Table 1: Old and new actors of calcium homeostasis.

Old actors	New actors
PTH	FGF 23
Calcitonin	TRPV5
Vitamin D	Klotho gene
Diet	
Physical exercise	
Ultra-violet exposition	

The gene FGF-23, a member of the fibroblast growth factor (FGF) family, and Klotho are also essential for the regulation of calcium metabolism [2]. FGF-23 gene is overexpressed in tumors causing cancer-induced osteomalacia, while Klotho gene deletion interferes with synthesis of bone matrix and spatial distribution of osteocytes [3, 4].

Transforming growth factor-beta (TGF-β), tumor necrosis factor (TNF), and interleukin-1 (IL-1) influence calcium metabolism exclusively in patients with malignancy-associated hypercalcemia (MAH) (see Chapter 3).

Physiologically, the parathyroid chief cells respond to a reduction of extracellular calcium by increasing secretion of PTH, at a rate inversely related to serum ionized calcium, according to a negative feed-back mechanism. In patients with primary HPT there is an excessive secretion of PTH, and loss of suppressive effect of extracellular calcium on parathyroid cells. The action of high serum PTH levels on target organs leads to hypercalcemia (see Chapter 1). Several other conditions should be considered as able to modify calcium levels (Table **2**).

Table 2: Conditions modifying calcium levels. UFCa = ultra filtrate calcium.

Cond-ition	Calcium serum level	UFCa	Bind protein
Hemoconcentration	↑	↔	↔
Hypherglobulinemia	↔↑	↑	↓
Serum protein > 5 g/L	↓	↔	↔
Serum protein < 5 g/L	↑ ↔ ↓	↑	↓
Acidosis pH < 7.3	↔	↑	↓
Alcalosis pH > 7.6	↔	↑	↑

PRIMARY HYPERPARATHYROIDISM: INCIDENCE, ETIOLOGY & PATHOGENESIS

The incidence of primary HPT is approximately 42 per 100,000, while in women aged over 60 years its prevalence is up to 4 per 1000 [5]. Sporadic primary HPT is caused by a solitary adenoma in 80-85%, multiglandular disease (multiple adenoma, parathyroid hyperplasia) in 12-14%, and a parathyroid carcinoma in 1-2% of the cases. Primary HPT can also occur in familial syndromes, such as (1) multiple endocrine neoplasia type 1 (MEN 1), (2) MEN type 2A (MEN 2A), (3) hyperparathyroidism-jaw tumor (HPT-JT) syndrome, and (4) familial isolated primary HPT (FIPH), which seems to be an early stage of MEN 1 or HPT-JT (Fig. **1**).

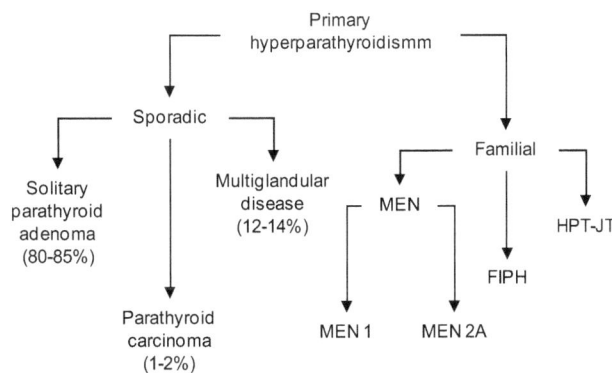

Figure 1: Causes of primary hyperparathyroidism. HPH-JT = hyperparathyroidism-jaw tumor, FIPH = familial isolated primary hyperparathyroidism, MEN = multiple endocrine neoplasia.

The main action of an excess of PTH is the stimulation of both osteoclastic and osteoblastic activity, with a prevalence of osteoclast activity. The increase of bone turnover leads to osteopenia or osteoporosis, and subsequent increases in serum calcium levels [6]. Thus, in patients with primary HPT excessive demineralization and weakening of bone are observed, resulting in an abnormal cortical porosity and cortical bone loss. In untreated patients with severe HPT, bone pain and pathologic fractures may also occur. The classic features of hyperparathyroid bone disease (*osteitis fibrosa cystica*) are subperiosteal resorption of cortical bone, coexisting areas of increased bone density and demineralization, bone cysts, and brown tumors. [5].

Chronic hypercalcemia may result in kidney stones and several other consequences, such as increasing risk of vascular and myocardial diseases. However, a direct relationship between serum calcium, PTH, and arterial blood pressure has been excluded [7, 8].

Parathyroid carcinoma is an uncommon finding, but a relatively higher incidence has been reported in Japan and Italy [9, 10]. The etiology of this tumor remains unclear. Multiple risk factors, including neck irradiation, end-stage renal disease, MEN and HPT-JT syndromes have been suggested [11].

Recent molecular analysis studies have hypothesized about the involvement of mutations of several genes in the pathogenesis of parathyroid cancer. It includes the oncogene cyclin D1 or parathyroid adenoma 1 (PRAD1), located at the chromosome 13, the retinoblastoma tumor suppressor (RB gene), and the p53 tumor suppressor [12]. There is increasing evidence that loss of hyperparathyroidism 2 (HRPT2) gene expression (aberrant methylation) is strongly associated with parathyroid carcinoma, kidney tumors and HPT-JT syndrome [13, 14]. Specific tumor suppressor genes such as HRPT2 have demonstrated loss of heterozygosity in up to 50% of parathyroid carcinomas [15].

CLINICAL FEATURES & DIAGNOSIS OF PRIMARY HYPERPARATHYROIDISM

The most part of patients with primary HPT (80-90%) are discovered because of asymptomatic hypercalcemia. Some patients, however, are diagnosed because of a high index of suspicion, such as bone mineral density (BMD) alterations (i.e. osteopenia) or unjustified recurrent bilateral nephrolithiasis. Virtually, all patients with primary HPT can be discovered by simultaneous increase of both serum calcium and PTH levels, and thus the diagnosis can be obtained by inclusion rather than by excluding all the other causes of hypercalcemia (Figs. **2** and **3**).

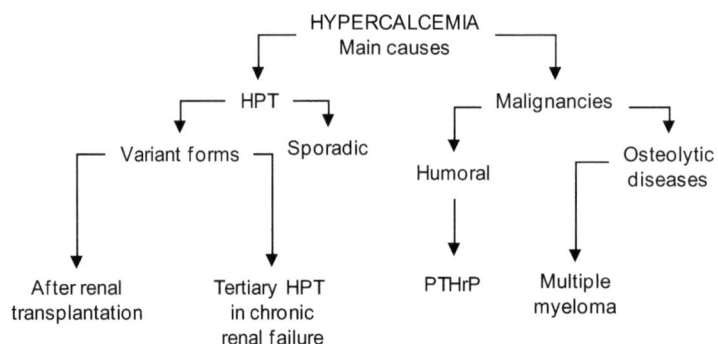

Figure 2: Main causes of hypercalcemia. HPT = hyperparathyroidism, PTH = parathyroid hormone. Modified from [5].

To obtain the "true" hypercalcemia, total serum calcium should be adjusted for the serum albumin concentration, and other confounding laboratory data should also be considered (see Chapter 5).

Moreover, most patients with nephrolithiasis and primary HPT may have intermittent hypercalcemia, so that more than one blood sample for serum calcium measurement should be obtained (see Chapter 1).

Occasionally, normocalcemic primary HPT may occur in patients with kidney stones or other problems. The main causes are: (1) hypoalbuminemia, (2) vitamin D deficiency, (3) increased phosphate intake, or (4) renal failure.

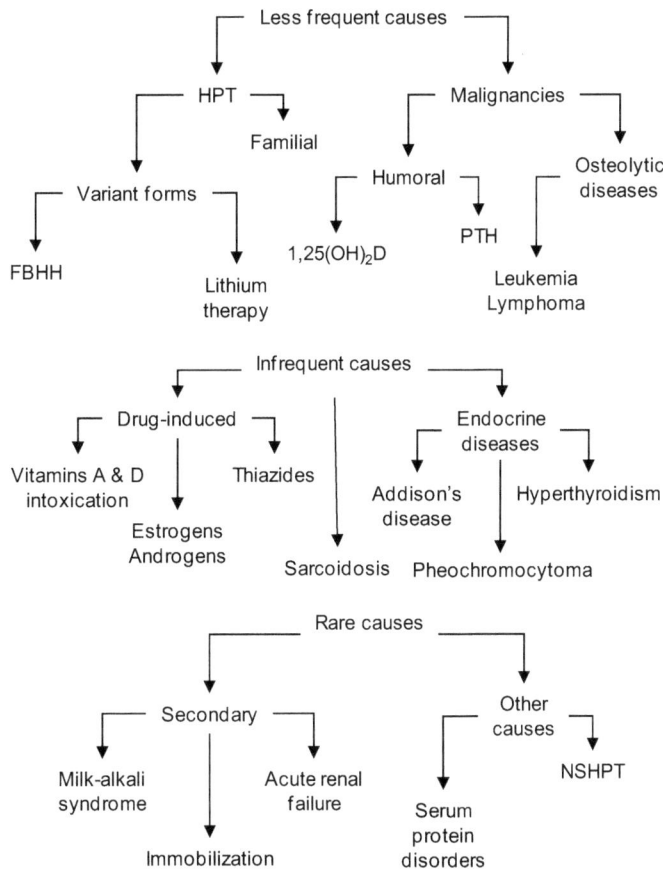

Figure 3: Less frequent and rare causes of hypercalcemia. HPT = hyperparathyroidism, PTH = parathyroid hormone, FBHH = familial benign hypocalciuric hypercalcemia, $1,25(OH)_2D = 1,25(OH)_2$ vitamin D (calcitriol). Modified from [5].

Patients with high PTH levels have unlikely other causes of hypercalcemia than primary HPT. The relationship between serum calcium and PTH in patients with primary HPT, MAH, and other diseases leading to changes of calcium metabolism are shown in Fig. **4**.

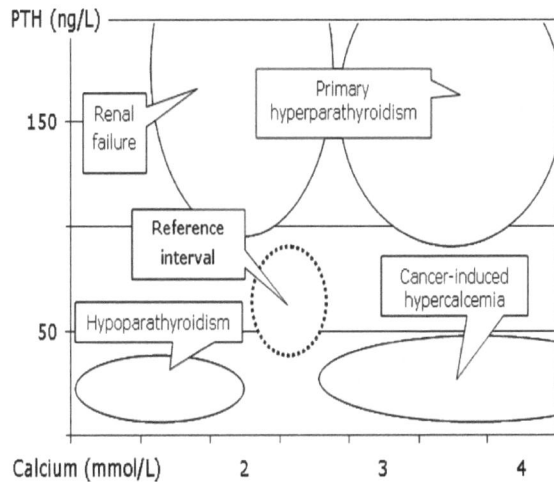

Figure 4: Relationship between serum calcium and parathyroid hormone (PTH) in patients with primary hyperparathyroidism, cancer-induced hypercalcemia and other diseases.

Usually, the first step of diagnosis is differentiating between primary HPT and MAH (Table **3**). Unfortunately, both signs and symptoms of primary HPT are usually nonspecific, mainly depending on serum calcium concentration. In patients with calcium serum level > 3 mmol/L, nausea, anorexia, thirst, vomiting, and polyuria can be observed. Whereas in those with hypercalcemia > 4 mmol/L, impairment of the conscious level usually occurs [17, 18].

Table 3: Laboratory findings for differential diagnosis between primary hyperparathyroidism and malignancy-associated hypercalcemia. PTH = parathyroid hormone, PTHrP = parathyroid hormone-related protein. Modified from [16].

Disease	Serum calcium	PTH	Calciuria	PTHrP
Primary hyperparathytoidism	< 12,5 mg/dL (< 3.13 mmol/L)	High-normal or elevated	High	Very low (< 2 pmol/L)
Malignancy-associated hypercalcemia	> 12,5 mg/dL (> 3.13 mmol/L)	Very low (< 20 ng/L)	Very high	High

The main signs and symptoms of patients with symptomatic primary HPT are shown in Fig. **5**.

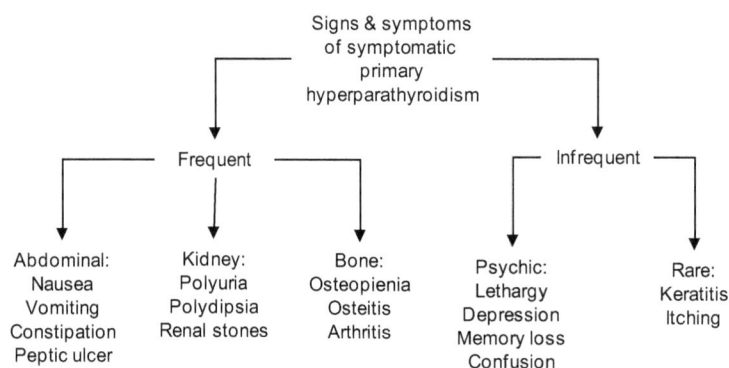

Figure 5: Main signs and symptoms in symptomatic patients with primary hyperparathyroidism. Modified form [5].

Virtually, all patients with confirmed symptomatic primary HPT should be referred for surgery. Several studies have demonstrated that after parathyroidectomy both BMD and cognitive function improve, fracture rate and incidence of kidney stones decline, and premature death due to cardiovascular disease appears to decrease [19]. Surgery should be considered for all patients with loss of bone density, and particularly in premenopausal women in which the improvement of BMD after parathyroidectomy is greater than in men. This suggests the need of endogenous estrogens for complete bone recovery [20]. In patients with persistent or recurrent primary HPT the histology of the removed parathyroid glands should be reviewed, and the biochemical diagnosis should be reconfirmed before any further surgical procedure (see Chapter 7).

In 1991 a NIH consensus conference stated that preoperative imaging was rarely used in patients with primary HPT. Furthermore, it had not proven to be cost effective, and did not shorten surgical time [21]. However, sensitivity of noninvasive localization techniques has improved significantly in the last decade, especially in patients with solitary parathyroid adenoma [22, 23].

Currently, the combination of ^{99m}Tc-sestamibi scintigraphy and high-resolution neck ultrasonography represents a reliable noninvasive procedure which, in conjunction with intraoperative quick-PTH assay, should be considered for use in each patient undergoing surgery for primary HPT [24, 25] (see Chapters 5 and 6). Fig. **6** shows a sestamibi scan image localizing a left inferior parathyroid adenoma.

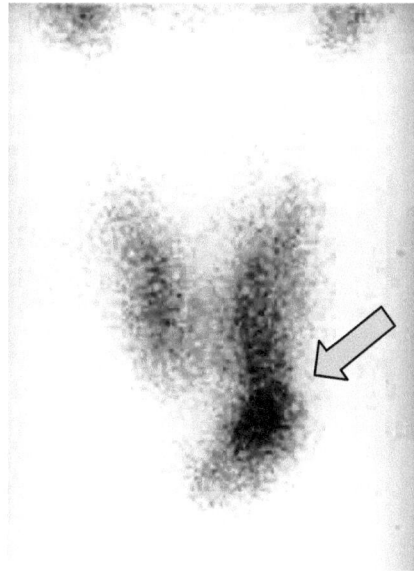

Figure 6: Parathyroid scan image obtained in a 57-year-old women with primary hyperparathyroidism due to a parathyroid adenoma of the left inferior parathyroid gland (arrow). Dual-isotope parathyroid scintigraphy is usually carried out using a single head gamma camera, equipped with a low-energy, parallel-hole high-resolution collimator. Patients are injected with 370 MBq ^{99m}Tc-methoxyisobutyl-isonitrile (sesta-mibi), and planar images of head, neck, and mediastinum are obtained (anterior view, matrix 256 x 256, 10-15 min per view). More images are acquired after 150 MBq ^{99m}Tc-pertechnetate administration.

Dual-phase scintigraphy is performed using a single tracer (sestamibi), acquiring images at 30 and 120 min. Positive scan is defined as a relative increased sestamibi uptake area persisting after images subtraction, or after the washout period [22, 24].

Thanks to these results, together with the development of minimally-invasive techniques, parathyroidectomy has become a surgical procedure commonly performed as a one-day surgery as well as being equally successful with outpatients [26]. Several studies have shown that the surgical treatment is cost-effective as compared with a medical monitoring strategy. Thus, improving the quality of life both in mild symptomatic patients and in those with asymptomatic primary HPT [1, 27] (see Chapter 7).

A 2008 workshop has defined new guidelines for parathyroidectomy in patients with asymptomatic primary HPT, that includes: (1) age <50 years, (2) serum calcium more than 0.25 mmol/L above the upper limits of normal, (3) estimated glomerular filtration ratio (eGFR) reduced to 60 mL/min, and (4) a BMD measured by osteodensitometry >2.5 standard deviations below the young normal mean (T-score) at any site [28]. Bone formation markers, such as bone specific alkaline phosphatase and osteocalcin are not useful in monitoring patients [29]. Some physicians still consider hypercalciuria (>10 mmol/L/24h) as an indicator for parathyroidectomy, according to 2002 Workshop guidelines, suggesting surgery also in patients for which medical surveillance is neither desirable nor possible [28, 30]. Familial isolated primary HPT (FIPH) is an autosomical dominant disorder, representing an early stage of either HPT-JT or MEN 1 syndromes. This condition can also be caused by an allelic variant of MEN 1 or HRPT2 genes, or by a distinct entity involving another locus [31]. Fig. 7 shows a flow-chart for diagnosing familial primary HPT.

Germline mutations in the MEN1 gene predispose to MEN 1 syndrome, but in up to 20-25% of clinical MEN 1 cases, no MEN1 mutations can be found [33]. A DNA test for MEN1 germline mutations is a useful tool for diagnosing MEN 1 (see Chapter 5). Thus, a subset of patients carry germline mutations in genes MEN1, HRPT2 and calcium-sensing receptor (CASR), predisposing them to syndromic forms of primary HPT or FIHP [34].

Familial primary hyperparathyroidism

↓

Search for other tumors in index patient
and in first-degree relatives

Pituitary
and GEP
tumors

MTC
Pheochromocytoma

Jaw tumor
Renal cysts
Wilms' tumor

No other tumor

FIPHP

Genetic test
for mutation of

MEN 1 → MEN 1

RET → MEN 2A

HRPT 2 → HPT-JT

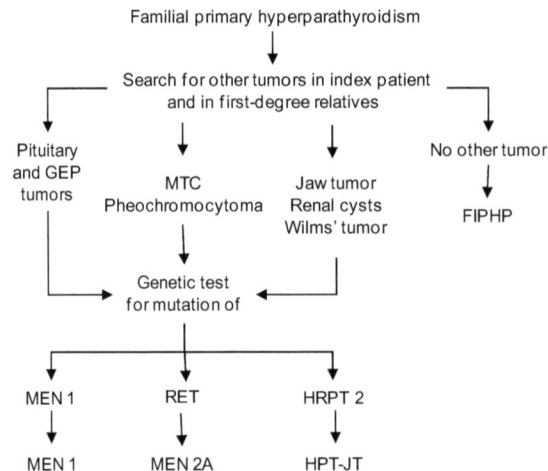

Figure 7: Diagnosing familial primary hyperparathyroidism. GEP = gastro-entero-pancreatic, MTC = medullary thyroid carcinoma, FIPHP = familial isolated primary hyperparathyroidism, HPT-JT = hyperparathyroidism-jaw tumor, MEN 1 = multiple endocrine neoplasia type 1, MEN 2A = multiple endocrine neoplasia type 2A. Modified from [32].

Recently, germline mutations in two novel genes, such as aryl hydrocarbon receptor-interacting protein (AIP), and cyclin-dependent kinase inhibitor 1B (CDKN1B), encoding p27 cyclin-dependent kinase inhibitor (Kip1), have been found to be associated with various endocrine tumors, including parathyroid tumors [34]. Although germline mutations in the CDKN1B gene is a rare cause of MEN 1, patients with this mutation may be predisposed to a MEN 1-like condition.

Most patients with refractory secondary or tertiary HPT have monoclonal parathyroid tumors, and inactivating mutations of CDKN1B were reported to cause HPT in MEN 1-like syndrome [35]. Table **4** reports criteria for differential diagnosis between sporadic primary HPT, familial HPT, familial benign hypocalciuric hypercalcemia (FBHH), and neonatal severe primary HPT (NSHPT).

Table 4: Differences between sporadic hyperparathyroidism (HPT), familial HPT, familial benign hypocalciuric hypercalcemia (FBHH), and neonatal severe primary HPT (NSHPT). PTH = parathyroid hormone. Median (range) values for age, serum calcium and PTH; frequency (%) for osteoporosis and kidney stones. Modified from [32].

DISEASE	Age (years)	Total serum calcium (mmol/L)	Serum PTH (pg/mL)	Osteoporosis (frequency)	Kidney stones (frequency)
Sporadic Hyperparathyroidism	63 (31-93)	2.78 (2.41-4.36)	137 (69-1301)	60.2%	43.1%
Familial Hyperparathyroidism	26 (12-74)	2.79 (2.57-3.36)	174 (84-414)	66%	40%
FBHH/NSHPT Syndromes	4 (0.1-26)	2.91 (2.84-3.30)	43.5 (34-56)	0%	0%

OTHER BENIGN DISEASES

Familial benign hypocalciuric hypercalcemia is a rare autosomal dominant disease reflecting partial resistance to the normal effects of extracellular calcium on parathyroid glands and kidneys. Homozygous loss-of-function CASR mutations manifest as NSHPT, a rare disorder characterized by extreme hypercalcemia and the bone changes of hyperparathyroidism, which occur in infancy [36].

FBHH is caused by heterozygous loss-of-function mutations in the CASR, and is responsible for asymptomatic mild hypercalcema accompanied by normal or slightly elevated PTH serum levels, and urinary calcium usually < 12.5 mmol/24 h. To better understand the mutations causing defects in the CASR gene and to define specific regions relevant for ligand-receptor interaction and other receptor functions, the data on mutations was collected and the information was centralized in the CASR database (www.casrdb.mcgill.ca) [36].

Up to 10% of patients with sarcoidisis may have hypercalciuria and hypercalcemia, due to inappropriate serum levels of 1,25(OH)$_2$ vitamin D [1,25(OH)$_2$D], while 25(OH) vitamin D [25(OH)D] is normal. The clinical features of sarcoidosis depends on the degree and site of tissue involvement, frequently the diagnosis is no more than an incidental radiological finding, and ultimately depends on results of biopsy. The activity of 25(OH)D 1-hydroxylase in lymphoid tissues of patients with sarcoidosis is elevated, and steroid administration normalizes both serum 1,25(OH)$_2$D and calcium levels.

Hypercalcemia is found also in 10% of patients with hyperthyroidism or thyrotoxicosis, and in those with Addison's disease, together with low PTH serum levels. Clinical manifestations of MEN 2A syndrome, an autosomal dominant disorder, include medullary thyroid carcinoma (80-100%), pheocromocytoma (40%) and HPT (25%) [37]. Indeed, hypercalcemia may be found in patients with MEN 2A, and also in patients with sporadic pheocromocytoma, due to increased parathyroid hormone-related protein (PTHrP) secreted by the tumor.

Increase of bone resorption, typically present in immobilized patients, may lead to hypercalcemia and PTH suppression. Milk-alkali syndrome is still seen occasionally. It is due to excess of ingestion of both alkali and calcium (in form of milk) to treat symptomatically peptic ulcer disease.

Rhabdomyolysis, usually observed in patients with acute renal failure, results in mobilization of calcium from muscle tissue, and subsequently hypercalcemia. The relationship between renal function, calcium metabolism, and posttransplant hyperparathyroidism, as well as the effects of thiazide diuretics and vitamin D intoxication, are discussed in Chapter 1.

CONCLUSIONS

Primary HPT and MAH are the most common causes of hypercalcemia. MAH is observed in up to 30% of cancer patients, especially in those with solid tumors and multiple myeloma. The differential diagnosis can be obtained by determining intact-PTH level. The 25(OH)D serum levels is often reduced in patients with primary HPT and may by a cause of normocalcemic primary HPT, while patients with MAH have usually a critical (>3.5 mmol/L) hypercalcemia.

MEN syndromes, FBHH, and lithium therapy should be considered as variants of primary HPT, showing specific laboratory findings. Several other causes of hypercalcemia, such as drug intoxication, renal failure, endocrine diseases, are easily distinguished from both primary HPT and MAH. Imaging studies are not required before biochemical diagnosis of primary HPT or MAH is confirmed.

REFERENCES

[1]   Zanocco K, Angelos P, Sturgeon C. Cost-effectiveness analysis of parathyroidectomy for symptomatic primary hyperparathyroidism. Surgery 2006; 140: 874-882.

[2]   Medici D, Razzaque MS, DeLuca S, *et al*. FGF-23-Klotho signaling stimulates proliferation and prevents vitamin D-induced apoptosis. J Cell Biol 2008; 182: 459-465.

[3]   Gkika D, Mahieu F, Nilius B, Hoenderop JG, Bindels RJ. 80K-H as a new Ca2+ sensor regulating the activity of the epithelial Ca2+ channel transient receptor potential cation channel V5 (TRPV5). J Biol Chem 2004; 279: 26351-26357.

[4]   Suzuki H, Amizuka N, Oda K, *et al*. Histological evidence of the altered distribution of osteocytes and bone matrix synthesis in Klotho-deficient mice. Arch Histol Cytol 2005; 68: 371-381.

[5]   Shoback D, Marcus R, Bikle D, Strewler G. Mineral metabolism & metabolic bone disease. In: Greenspan FS & Gardner DG, Eds. Basic & Clinical Endocrinology. New York, Lange Medical Books/McGraw Hill, 2001; pp. 237-333.

[6] Christiansen P. The skeleton in primary hyperparathyroidism: a review focusing on bone remodeling, structure, mass, and fracture. APIMIS Suppl. 2001; 102: 1-52.

[7] Lumachi F, Ermani M, Luisetto G, *et al*. Relationship between serum parathyroid hormone, serum calcium and arterial blood pressure in patients with primary hyperparathyroidism: results of a multivariate analysis. Eur J Endocrinol 2002; 146: 643-647.

[8] Lumachi F, Ermani M, Frego M, *et al*. Intima-media thickness measurement of the carotid artery in patients with primary hyperparathyroidism. A prospective case-control study and long-term follow-up. In Vivo 2006; 20: 887-890.

[9] Lumachi F, Ermani M, Marino F, *et al*. Relationship of AgNOR counts and nuclear DNA content to survival in patients with parathyroid carcinoma. Endocr Relat Cancer 2004; 11: 563-569.

[10] Lumachi F, Basso SMM, Basso U. Parathyroid cancer. Etiology, clinical presentation and treatment. Anticancer Res 2006; 26: 4803-4808.

[11] Rawat N, Khetan N, Williams DW, *et al*. Parathyroid carcinoma. Br J Surg 2005; 92: 1345-1353, 2005.

[12] Shane E. Clinical review 122: parathyroid carcinoma. J Clin Endocrinol Metab 2001; 86: 485-493.

[13] Hewitt KM, Sharma PK, Samowitz W, Hobbs M. Aberrant methylation of HRPT2 gene in parathyroid carcinoma. Ann Otol Rhinol Laryngol 2007; 116: 928-933.

[14] Hahn MA, McDonnell J, Marsh DJ. The effect of disease-associated HRPT2 mutations on splicing. J Endocrinol 2009; 201: 387-396.

[15] Yip L, Seethala RR, Nikiforova MN, *et al*. Loss of heterozygosity of selected tumor suppressor genes in parathyroid carcinoma. Surgery 2008; 144: 949-955.

[16] Toffaletti JG. Blood gasses and electrolytes. 2nd Ed. Washington, DC: AACC Press; 2009.

[17] Heath DA. Hypercalcemia of malignancy. In: Russell RGG & Kanis JA (Eds), Tumor-induced hypercalcemia and its management. Royal Society of Medicine, London, 1991: 29-31.

[18] Lumachi F, Brunello A, Roma A, Basso U. Cancer-induced hypercalcemia. Anticancer Res 2009: 29: 1551-1556.

[19] Udelsman R, Pasieka JL, Sturgeon C, Young JEM, Clark OH. Surgery for Asymptomatic primary hyperparathyroidism: proceedings of the third international workshop. J Clin Endocrinol Metab 2009; 94: 366-372.

[20] Lumachi F, Camozzi V, Ermani M, De Lotto F, Luisetto G. Bone mineral density improvement after successful parathyroidectomy in pre- and postmenopausal women with primary hyperparathyroidism. Ann N Y Acad Sci 2007; 1117: 357-361.

[21] NIH Conference. Diagnosis and management of asymptomatic primary hyperparathyroidism. Consensus development conference statement. Ann Intern Med 1991; 114: 593-597.

[22] Lumachi F, Ermani M, Basso S, *et al*. Localization of parathyroid tumours in the minimally invasive era: which technique should be chosen ? Population-based analysis of 253 patients undergoing parathyroidectomy and factors affecting parathyroid gland detection. Endocr Relat Cancer 2001; 8: 63-69.

[23] Mihai R, Simon D, Hellman P. Imaging for primary hyperparathyroidism. An evidence-based analysis. Langenbecks Arch Surg 2009; 394: 765-784.

[24] Lumachi F, Zucchetta P, Marzola MC, *et al*. Advantages of combined technetium-99m-sestamibi scintigraphy and high-resolution ultrasonography in parathyroid localization: comparative study in 91 patients with primary hyperparathyroidism. Eur J Endocrinol 2000; 143: 755-760.

[25] Irvin GL, Carneiro DM. Intraoperative parathyroid hormone assay as a surgical adjunct in patients with sporadic primary hyperparathyroidism. In: Clark OH, Duh Q-Y, Kebebew E, Eds. Textbook of Endocrine surgery. Philadelphia, Elvevier Saunders, 2005; pp. 472-480.

[26] Grant CS, Thompson G, Farley D, van Heerden J. Primary hyperparathyroidism surgical management since the introduction of minimally invasive parathyroidectomy. Mayo Clinic experience. Arch Surg 2005; 140: 472-478.

[27] Sheldon DG, Lee FT, Neil NJ, Ryan JA Jr. Surgical treatment of hyperparathyroidism improves health-related quality of life. Arch Surg 2002; 137:1022-1026.

[28] Bilezikian JP, Khan AA, Potts JT. Guidelines for the management of asymptomatic Primary Hyperparathyroidism: summary statement from the Third International Workshop. J Clin Endocrinol Metab 2009; 94: 335-339.

[29] Lumachi F, Ermani M, Camozzi V, Tombolan V, Luisetto G. Changes of bone formation markers osteocalcin and bone-specific alkaline phosphatase in postmenopausal women with osteoporosis. Ann N Y Acad Sci 2009; 1173: E60-E63.

[30] Bilezikian JP, Potts JT Jr, Fuleihan GEH, *et al.* Summary statement from a Workshop on asymptomatic Primary Hyperparathyroidism: a perspective for the 21st century. J Clin Endocrinol Metab 2002; 87: 5353-5361.

[31] Hannan FM, Nesbit MA, Christie PT, *et al.* Familial isolated primary hyperparathyroidism caused by mutations of the MEN1 gene. Nat Clin Pract Endocrinol Metab 2008; 4: 53-58.

[32] Töke J, Patócs A, Balogh K, *et al.* Parathyroid hormone-dependent hypercalcemia. Wien Klin Wochenschhr 2009; 121: 236-245.

[33] Georgitsi M, Raitila A, Karhu A, van der Luijt RB, *et al.* Germline CDKN1B/p27Kip1 mutation in multiple endocrine neoplasia. J Clin Endocrinol Metab 2007; 92: 3321-3325.

[34] Vierimaa O, Villablanca A, Alimov A, *et al.* Mutation analysis of MEN1, HRPT2, CASR, CDKN1B and AIP genes in primary hyperparathyroidism patients with features of genetic predisposition. J Endocrinol Invest 2009; PMID: 19474519.

[35] Lauter KB, Arnold A. Mutational analysis of CDKN1B, a candidate tumor-suppressor gene, in refractory secondary/tertiary hyperparathyroidism. Kidney Int 2008; 73: 1137-1140.

[36] Pidasheva S, D'Souza-Li L, Canaff L, Cole DE, Hendy GN. CASRdb: calcium-sensing receptor locus-specific database for mutations causing familial (benign) hypocalciuric hypercalcemia, neonatal severe hyperparathyroidism, and autosomal dominant hypocalcemia. Hum Mutat 200; 24: 107-111.

[37] Gardner DG. Multiple endocrine neoplasia. In: Greenspan FS & Gardner DG, Eds. Basic & Clinical Endocrinology. New York, Lange Medical Books/McGraw Hill, 2001; pp. 792-801.

CHAPTER 3

Hypercalcemia and Malignancy

Umberto Basso, Anna Roma and Antonella Brunello

Istituto Oncologico Veneto (IOV) IRCCS, 35128 Padova, Italy

Abstract: Hypercalcemia arising in cancer patients is usually referred to as malignancy-associated hypercalcemia (MAH). It may complicate early or, more often, late phases of the disease with a prevalence of around 5-30% of all patients with different types of cancer. However, the prophylactic use of bisphosphonates to prevent skeletal events in patients with bone metastases, has probably reduced the occurrence of clinically symptomatic MAH. The most frequent cause of MAH is abnormal production of a parathyroid hormone-related protein (PTHrP), which mimics the effects of parathyroid hormone, increasing bone resorption and, especially, renal tubular calcium reabsorption. Other causes may be bone lysis due to several cytokines and mediators released by the cancer cells in the bone or the ectopic production of $1,25(OH)_2$ vitamin D_3 in tumor tissue. Periodical monitoring of serum ions in cancer patients usually unveils the onset of MAH before the appearance of the classical symptoms (headache, confusion, de-hydration), prompting adequate treatment consisting in hydration, diuretics, bisphosphonates and, whenever possible, treatment of the underlying cancer (usually with systemic chemotherapy). Bisphosphonates are a class of compounds which have all shown to decrease serum calcium levels primarily by inhibition of PTH-dependent osteoclast activation. Although, the antiresorptive potency is higher with late generation compounds (pamidronate, zolendronate, ibandronate) compared to older oral compounds. Agents able to interfere with the receptor activator of nuclear actor-κ ligand (RANKL) pathway such as the monoclonal antibody denosumab represent novel and promising strategies for the treatment of MAH which are currently undergoing experimental and clinical assessment.

INTRODUCTION

Hypercalcemia developing in patients with primary or metastatic cancer is named malignancy-associated hypercalcemia (MAH) and arises in around 3% to 30% of all cancer patients [1, 2]. MAH develops mainly in patients affected by lung (especially those with squamous histology), breast, head & neck, kidney & urinary tract cancer, as well as in multiple myeloma. However, it is relatively rare in gastrointestinal and prostate cancer and almost absent in primary bone tumors (Table **1**). Establishing an actual incidence rate is difficult due to the differences in the natural history and impact of treatments on tumors, the heterogeneity of cut-off levels for calcium measurement applied in different studies (total or albumin-corrected) and the inclusion of asymptomatic cases. Moreover, it has been speculated that the widespread use of bisphosphonates administered prophylactically to patients with bone metastases in order to prevent skeletal events probably allows to avoid and/or reduce the intensity of hypercalcemic events [1].

Table 1: Primary site of cancer causing malignancy-associated hypercalcemia (MAH).

Frequent onset of MAH (10-30%)	MAH rather infrequent (<10%)	MAH extremely rare (1% or less)
Multiple myeloma Lung cancer Breast cancer Kidney-cancer Parathyroid cancer Adult T-cell leukemia	Gastro-esophageal cancer Colorectal cancer Prostate cancer Lymphoma	Osteosarcoma Soft tissue sarcomas Melanoma

It is usually believed that the frequency and severity of MAH are higher in patients with lytic bone lesions compared to those with osteoblastic alterations due to the hypothesis that calcium might remain entrapped within the bone. This might explain the low incidence of MAH in patients with prostate cancer despite a high incidence of bone involvement, although others factors (such as PSA-mediated cleavage of hypercalcemic mediators) might be implicated. Malignancy-associated hypercalcemia is usually found in patients with advanced tumors after several treatments thus explaining a short survival usually in the range of a few months. At the same time, cases of MAH arising at the initial diagnosis in chemosensitive tumors (especially multiple myeloma or metastatic breast cancer) may still obtain long-term remissions [3]. Yet, it is noteworthy to mention that even asymptomatic calcium elevation in patients with prostate cancer may be associated with increased risk of skeletal events and death [4].

ETIOLOGY & PATHOPHYSIOLOGY

Physiologically, elevation of serum calcium depends upon mobilization of bone reserves, inhibition of renal tubular excretion and increased bowel absorption. All of these three events have been found to sustain MAH according to three main mechanisms (Table **2**):

- Production of parathyroid hormone-related protein (PTHrP) and, much less frequently, parathyroid hormone (PTH) itself, acting on bone and kidney;

- Ectopic activation of vitamin D to 1,25-dihydroxy vitamin D [$1,25(OH)_2D$] with increases bowel absorption of calcium and minor effects on bone and kidney;

- Bone lysis induced by cancer cells which, after invading the bone, promotes degradation of mineral matrix.

Table 2: Types of malignancy-associated hypercalcemia (MAH). PTH = parathyroid hormone, PTHrP = parathyroid hormone-related protein, $1,25(OH)_2D_3$ = 1,25-dihydroxy vitamin D_3.Modified from [2].

Type	Frequency	Bone metastases	Causal agent	Typical tumors
Local osteolytic MAH	20%	Present	Cytokines PTHrP	Breast cancer multiple myeloma lymphoma/leukemia lung cancer kidney cancer
Humoral MAH	80%	Present or absent	PTHrP	Squamous-cell cancer (i.e. head and neck, lung) renal cancer ovarian cancer breast cancer endometrial cancer HTLV-associated lymphoma
Parathyroid carcinoma	<1%	Not rare	PTH	Parathyroid carcinoma
Ectopic PTH-secreting tumor	<1%	Variable	PTH	Variable
$1,25(OH)_2D_3$ -secreting cancer	<1%	Variable	$1,25(OH)_2D_3$	Lymphoma (all types) Some solid tumors

Parathyroid hormone-related protein-dependent hypercalcemia is usually termed "humoral MAH" in the sense that it does not require direct bone involvement by tumor cells, while the presence of bone metastases is a pre-requisite for the osteolytic mechanism. Since production of PTHrP and bone lysis often coexist in the same patient with MAH, the extent of bone involvement may not be correlated with the severity of hypercalcemia. On the contrary, increased intestinal calcium absorption has usually a marginal role in MAH, although some exceptions have been documented.

Parathyroid Hormone-related Protein

Since the early 1940s it was speculated that elevation of serum calcium in patients with cancer might be related to some "humoral" agent produced by the tumor, which was able to induce hypercalcemia even in the absence of bone involvement.

PTH is responsible for hypercalcemia in patients with parathyroid adenoma or carcinoma and ectopic secretion has been found in some carcinomas. Subsequently, it was found that a peptide immunologically close but not coincident with PTH could be isolated from the blood and tumor biopsies of patients with MAH, therefore called PTHrP, which was able to induce hypercalcemia when injected in animals. Its gene was eventually cloned in 1987 [5].

Parathyroid hormone-related protein shares a sequence homology with PTH at the N-terminal aminoacid sequence, it has also unique sequences. Several biochemical studies demonstrated that PTHrP is able to bind to the same receptors of PTH (located mainly in the bone and the kidney) by means of the homologous N-terminal region as well as activating different pathways through interaction with specific receptors recognizing the non-homologous parts of the protein. These differences may explain why PTHrP has been found to exert its hypercalcemic action mainly in the kidney with less prominent effects on bone resorption and $1,25(OH)_2D$ generation compared to PTH [6].

For these reasons MAH may be sometimes refractory to antiresorptive agents despite the evidence of persistent suppression of bone resorption since they do not affect the inhibition of calcium excretion from the kidney [7]. Indeed, by alternating the splicing of the gene of PTHrP, it may generate various mRNA transcripts which are translated in slightly different peptides expressed also in normal tissues (such as skin keratinocytes, endocrine glands, central nervous system). Thus allowing the speculation of still poorly documented physiologic activities beyond the well-known induction of MAH in cancer patients as well as their possible involvement in fetal development of epithelial tissues and in the pathogenesis of some endocrine diseases as diabetes mellitus.

Several other agents have been shown to induce bone lysis and hypercalcemia in experimental models as well as in vivo such as interleukin 1 (IL-1), interleukin 6 (IL-6), transforming growth factor-alpha (TGF-α) and beta (TGF-β), tumor necrosis factor (TNF) and some growth factors. However their role as mediators of MAH is much less documented compared to PTHrP, which may be been found in up to 100% of blood samples of hypercalcemic cancer patients free from bone metastases [1]. At the same time, PTHrP expression studies by immunohistochemistry showed its presence in tumor tissues of both hypercalcemic and normocalcemic patients as a demonstration that complex gene expression mechanisms and several clinical factors may interfere with the developing of PTHrP dependent MAH.

Production of Active Metabolites of Vitamin D

In some patients with lymphomas, solid tumors or immunological disorders such as sarcoidosis, abnormal conversion of 25-hydroxyvitamin D $[25(OH)D_3]$ to $1,25(OH)_2D_3$ may increase intestinal absorption of calcium and cause hypercalcemia, usually less severe compared to PTHrP related cases. These cases may be identified by dosage of circulating $1,25(OH)_2D_3$ as well as by immunostaining for the $25(OH)_2D_3$ 1-alpha-hydroxylase. These cases sustain significant benefits from therapy with steroids which induce increased intestinal excretion of calcium [8].

Bone Lysis

Replacement of normal bone marrow by metastatic cancer cells or malignant leukocytes or plasma cells have two major consequences: depletion of normal blood cells and degradation of mineralized matrix ensuing in MAH. The bone in fact undergoes continuous remodeling by the opposite activities of bone forming osteoblasts and bone destroying osteoclasts. A complex interaction between tumor cells with stromal cells. The bone matrix creates the so called "vicious cycle" in which direct cell to cell interactions and local production of cytokines (IL-1, IL-6, TNF-α and TGF-β), chemokines and prostaglandins disrupt the normal balance in favor of bone resorption.

The receptor activator of nuclear actor-κ ligand (RANKL) system has recently been recognized as a central pathway leading to osteoclast differentiation and activation in MAH. These studies currently represent an exciting new target for the treatment of bone metastases [9]. RANKL is a TNF super-family trans-membrane protein which has been previously named as TNF-related activation-induced cytokine (TRANCE) or osteoclastic differentiation factor (ODF). RANKL has been found extensively expressed in bone and lymphoid tissues, but especially on the surface of activated osteoblasts after exposure to PTH, $1,25(OH)_2D_3$ or TNF-α. The receptor for RANKL is a protein expressed by osteoclast precursor cells of the monocyte-macrophage lineage and mature osteoclasts and dendritic cells. The RANK-RANKL interaction activates several intracellular pathways comprising nuclear factor-kappa (NF-κ), c-Jun N-terminus kinase (JNK) and p38 mitogen-activated protein tyrosine kinase (MAPK), and ultimately inducing differentiation, activation and survival of osteoclasts [10]. Tumor cells, circulating PTHrP but also several cytokines that are produced locally by normal bone marrow or stromal cells are principally responsible for a sustained activation of the RANKL cascade leading to MAH [11]. Fig. **1** resumes the interactions between osteoclasts and cancer-cells.

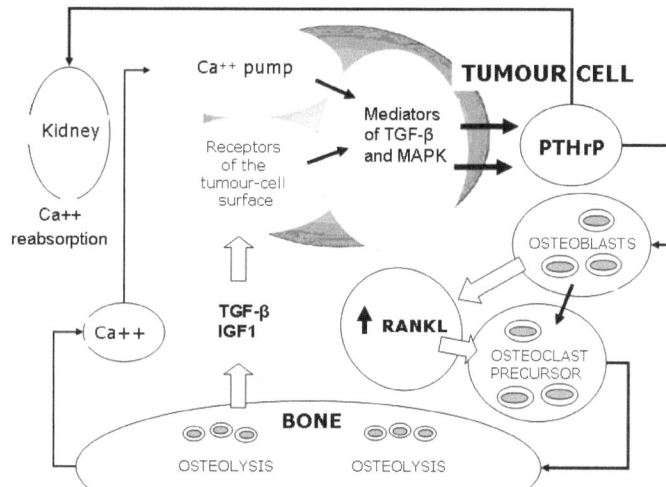

Figure 1: Interactions between osteoclasts and cancer-cells. PTHrP: parathyroid hormone-related protein, RANKL: receptor activator of nuclear factor-κ ligand, IGF: insulin-like growth factor, TGF-β: transforming growth factor-β, MAPK: mitogen-activated protein kinase. (Reproduced, with permission, from Lumachi F *et al.* Cancer-induced hypercalcemia. Anticancer Res 2009; 29: 1551-1556).

Osteoprotegerin (OPG) is another TNF superfamily member which, on the contrary, may serve as a soluble decoy receptor of RANKL and is able to inhibits its interaction with RANK. Inhibitors of RANKL and recombinant OPG may therefore be exploited as therapeutic tool for MAH (see below). In spite of the scientific evidence of the central role of RANKL system in bone pathology, clinical application of anti-RANKL therapy has just begun and there is a need of further clinical studies to uncover all its possible advantages in patients with acute MAH.

CLINICAL FEATURES

The clinical features of hypercalcemia are wide-ranging but usually non-specific (Table **3**) [12]. The severity of symptoms in the individual patient depends upon his general medical conditions, the ultimate level of plasma calcium as well as the rate of the ascent of calcium levels. Hypercalcemia in MAH is usually steadily and rapidly progressive and symptoms may develop at a lower plasma concentration than would be expected.

Since MAH often occurs in advanced phases of the disease, symptomatic deterioration may be wrongly attributed to progression of primary cancer, rather than elevation in serum calcium levels. Yet, recognizing signs and symptoms of hypercalcemia may have a much relevant impact on the quality of life of cancer patients since the condition is usually reversible with appropriate treatment and inturn rapid clinical improvements can be obtained [13]. Moreover, gastrointestinal manifestations such as anorexia, nausea and vomiting are early and common symptoms in hypercalcemic patients but can be erroneously attributed to the concomitant cytotoxic therapies.

Table 3: Symptoms & signs of malignancy-associated hypercalcemia (MAH).

Renal	Gastrointestinal	Central Nervous System	Cardiovascular
Polyuria Thirst Polydipsia Dehydration Renal failure Nephrocalcinosis Nephrolithiasis (rare in MAH)	Anorexia Nausea Vomiting Constipation Pancreatitis (rare in MAH)	Confusion Cognitive difficulties Coma Depression Ataxia Lethargy Psychosis Muscle weakness Fatigue	Hypertension Bradycardia ECG changes Orthostatic hypotension

Neurological manifestations can occur in a large part of patients, ranging from a slight confusion with mild cognitive difficulties and neuromuscular disturbances (muscle weakness, fatigue) to psychosis, ataxia, lethargy and lastly in coma. Older patients with pre-existing neurological or cognitive dysfunction may become severely obtunded even in the presence of mild hypercalcemia, whereas younger patients with moderate to severe hypercalcemia may not show any cognitive alteration.

Renal manifestations include polydipsia and polyuria with consequent dehydration that may further exacerbate hypercalcemia leading to renal failure. In general, the neurological and renal complications worsen with increasing severity of hypercalcemia. Patients may present also cardiologic symptoms such as hypertension and bradycardia and an electrocardiogram examination may show a shortened QT interval.

DIAGNOSIS

Most patients with mild hypercalcemia are asymptomatic and the condition is usually discovered as an incidental finding on routine standard laboratory tests which are periodically performed in the majority of cancer patients. Hypercalcemia may occasionally be the first sign of a multiple myeloma, or represent a paraneoplastic syndrome associated with occult solid cancer (usually in the presence of squamous-cell carcinoma of the tracheo-bronchial tract or upper gastro-esophageal system, clear-cell carcinoma of the kidney, hepatocarcinoma) [1, 3].

Parathyroid cancer is a rare occurrence, accounting for about 1% of cases of primary hyperparathyroidism, and patients usually have very high serum levels of PTH together with severe hypercalcemia [14, 15] (see Chapter 7).

Although clinical laboratories usually measure total serum calcium levels, the quantification of ionized calcium (the biologically active form) should be preferred, especially in patients with advanced metastatic cancer, because the decreases in albumin level are often related to malnutrition or hepatic failure. This may reduce total calcium values without altering the concentration of the ionized part.

Algorithms for calculation of albumin-corrected calcium have been proposed, although prospective validation of its utility is limited.

When calcium levels are elevated, differential diagnosis includes distinction of MAH from other benign causes, such as primary hyperparathyroidism, concomitant medications, and granulomatous diseases and then, if MAH is the cause, a further evaluation should analyze the pathogenetic mechanisms by which cancer increases calcium levels (Table **2**). The first step is the determination of plasma levels of the intact PTH. In patients with elevated or "inappropriately detectable" PTH, primary hyperparathyroidism is the most likely diagnosis (see Chapter 2). True ectopic PTH production is extremely rare in cancer patients (Table **2**), and the finding of an increased PTH level in a hypercalcemic patient with cancer is more likely to be due to a concomitant primary hyperparathyroidism [2]. In non-hyperparathyroid patients, the physiological response to hypercalcemia is the suppression of PTH secretion, with subsequent transitory reduction of both bone resorption and production of $1,25(OH)_2D_3$, and increase of calcium excretion. In patients with MAH, PTH serum levels are usually low, and the onset of the syndrome is usually anticipated by cancer-related symptoms, concomitant chemotherapy or analgesic therapies.

Quantification of circulating PTHrP in patients with MAH is feasible, yet guidelines for PTHrP testing in the clinical practice are still lacking, and since PTHrP levels do not change the treatment, the measurement may be proposed currently only for patients with controversial causes of hypercalcemia or for patients with MAH refractory to conventional treatment. Moreover, the inverse relationship with circulating PTH suggests that PTHrP should be tested only in patients with low levels of PTH [3,13,16] (see Chapter 5).

The assessment of serum creatinine, creatinine clearance and electrolytes is required to monitor renal function. Raised serum bicarbonate may suggest a calcium-alkali syndrome [13]. Electrocardiogram may be useful to recognize early rhythm disturbances induced by hypercalcemia. Plasma $1,25(OH)_2D_3$ should be measured when sarcoidosis, and other granulomatous disorders, or the $1,25(OH)_2D_3$ tumor syndrome are to be considered in the differential diagnosis [2] (see Chapter 2). If not previously performed, a bone scan is useful to assess the presence of bone metastases and the skeletal tumor burden in patients with cancer and hypercalcemia. Bone scintigraphy is usually positive long before the appearance of lytic alterations of routine x-rays. This is due to the persistence of some osteoblastic activity at the osteoclastic pit areas; yet, scintigraphy may be falsely negative in multiple myeloma or other occasional conditions of extensive bone resorption.

MEDICAL TREATMENT

Hydration with normal saline solution coupled with intravenous administration of bisphosphonates represent the standard treatment of MAH, although appropriate management and treatment of the underlying malignancy itself is crucial for an effective and durable clinical improvement.

Important general supportive measures that have to be adopted before the use of specific medications include an increase in the weight-bearing mobility of the patient, when possible. The discontinuation of calcium supplementation and concomitant treatments that can independently cause hypercalcemia, such as thiazide diuretics or lithium [2].

The second step consists in vigorous hydration with 0,9% saline solution, in order to restore intravascular volume, by increasing the filtered load of calcium through an increase of the glomerular filtration rate and to inhibit calcium reabsorption in the proximal nephron [2]. The rate of fluid replacement is determined by the serum calcium concentration, the severity of dehydration, and the patient's comorbidities such as renal or cardiac impairment [12]. After normovolemia has been reached, loop diuretics such as furosemide can be used to increase the renal excretion of calcium. The combination of furosemide and normal saline is seldom sufficient to treat hypercalcemia, because it reduces serum calcium levels only up to 15%, and enhanced diuresis may be complicated by iatrogenic electrolytes alterations [17].

Intravenous administration of bisposphonates is the treatment of first choice in the treatment of MAH because of their efficacy, relatively prolonged duration of action, and lack of acute toxicity [3,18]. All these compounds rapidly decrease calcium levels through inhibition of bone resorption with similar mechanisms comprising inhibition of osteoclasts and modulation of the activity of ostoblasts and macrophages. The effects on tubular calcium reabsorption in the kidney and $1,25(OH)_2D_3$ generation are marginally relevant (see Chapter 1). Most bisphosphonates, with the exception of clodronate and ibandronate, have a very low oral bioavailability, while after intravenous injection they are rapidly absorbed by the bone. Little toxicity has been described using bisphosphonates in the treatment of MAH. Etidronate and clodronate are currently considered drugs of second choice, due to their superior efficacy compared to other compounds [3].

Currently, the bisphosphonates recommended for the treatment of MAH are pamidronate, zoledronate or ibandronate. The administration of pamidronate over a 2-4 hour infusion, led to normocalcemia in more than 80% of patients, without significant renal toxicity [13,19]. Randomized trials have proved that pamidronate is superior to clodronate, etidronate, and mitramycin [18,19] but inferior to zoledronate in the rate and duration of control of MAH. Four mg of zoledronate is the recommended dose for initial treatment of MAH, while higher doses can be used in relapsing or refractory patients. The use of zoledronate is contraindicated if creatinine clearance is below 30 mL/min, and/or other nephrotoxic drugs are given to the patient [22] (see Chapter 8). A randomized trial showed a comparable activity of ibandronate and pamidronate in reducing calcium levels [23]. Ibandronate has an extremely favorable toxicity profile with very low rate of nephrotoxicity and can be safely used also in patients with moderate renal impairment [3]. Biochemical response to bisphosphonates is usually observed within 2-4 days and the nadir is reached within 7-10 days.

Normocalcemia, reached after the first dose in up to 90% of patients, is usually maintained for up to 3 weeks following treatment. A second dose can be administered 7-10 days after the first dose in patients in which serum calcium is persistently elevated [24]. Corticosteroids (i.e. prednisone) are sometimes employed to reduce intestinal calcium absorption and hypercalcemia-related nausea as well as to improve concomitant cancer-related symptoms. Although they are ineffective in the treatment of MAH with the exception of patients with multiple myeloma or lymphoma, in whom they have a direct antineoplastic activity or some patients with abnormally high bowel absorption, such those with excess of $1,25(OH)_2D_3$ [3].

Bisphosphonates do not alter the production of PTHrP by the malignancy, nor do these drugs affect the action of this molecule on the renal tubule. Higher levels of PTHrP can therefore predict an incomplete or poor response to bisphosphonates [17]. Other drugs were once used to treat MAH (i.e. mithramycin, gallium nitrate), but they are currently considered outdated options, with the only exception of calcitonin which may still constitute a safe treatment for refractory patients. This hormone physiologically intervenes in case of hypercalcemia counteracting the PTH actions on bone and kidney and was characterized by a rapid onset of action, limited incidence of side effects and absence of renal toxicity. Yet, reduction in serum calcium levels is usually low and receptor tachyphylaxis may appear rather early after treatment [17].

Calcitionin in combination with corticosteroids might be of particular relevance for patients with kidney failure unable to receive pamidronate or zolendronate, although the availability of non-nephrotoxic bisphosphonates such as ibandronate limits its clinical application [3].

Hypophosphatemia develops in most patients with hypercalcemia, but the use of oral or intravenous supplementation of phosphate is usually discouraged in clinical practice, since it can precipitate renal failure, induce seizures, abnormal cardiac conduction and diarrhea [2]. Dialysis with a low calcium dialysate may be useful in selected patient with hypercalcemia refractory to other treatments, especially when a chronic or acute renal failure is present [1, 13].

NEW TREATMENT APPROACHES TO MALIGNANCY-ASSOCIATED HYPERCALCEMIA

Different molecules have been proposed as novel treatments of MAH during the last years. The RANKL system represents the most promising target for the development of new treatments of MAH [2, 9]. The use of recombinant OPG, for example, inhibits the activity of RANKL and when administered to murine models, they both prevent MAH and reversed bone turnover, with a rapid normalization of calcium levels. In a recent study, OPG induced a more rapid effect on bone resorption compared to bisphosphonates in animal models of PTHrP-dependent MAH [7].

Another agent able to interfere with RANKL pathway is the fully human monoclonal antibody denosumab (AMG 162), which blocks RANKL-RANK interaction, mimicking the physiologic effects of OPG. The first studies with denosumab in postmenopausal osteoporotic women showed potent antiresorptive effect, with a dose-dependent, rapid and sustained decrease of bone turnover [25, 26]. Denosumab was also effective in inducing an early and sustained decrease of bone resorption in patients with multiple myeloma or breast cancer with bone metastases [27]. Recent clinical trials showed that denosumab suppresses bone resorption markers independently of prior bisphosphonates treatment and reduces skeletal events [28]. Anyway, the role of this agent in the acute management of MAH has still to be assessed (see Chapter 8).

PTHrP may be a potential target of treatment of MAH as well. A humanized antibody against PTHrP was tested in animal models of MAH, demonstrating its ability to completely normalize blood calcium level through an improvement of bone metabolism and calcium renal excretion, not affected by antiresorptive agents. This agent could be useful especially in patients developing bisphosphonate-refractory MAH [29, 30].

PROGNOSIS

MAH usually occurs in patients with advanced cancer and the finding of hypercalcemia in these subjects is a very poor prognostic factor, with a median survival of few months, 50% dying within 30 days. Furthermore, there is no definitive evidence that life-expectancy improves in patients who are actively treated for hypercalcemia, unless the underlying cancer is treatable with standard therapies. Raised serum levels of PTHrP indicate a reduced response to bisphosphonates, a more advanced tumor state and, therefore, a poorer prognosis [31].

For some tumors increased calcium is an independent prognostic factor for survival: hypercalcemia defined stage III in the well-known staging system of multiple myeloma proposed by Durie and Salmon, as well as it is still an item of the expanded Motzer criteria for current risk stratification of patients with metastatic renal cell carcinoma [32].

CONCLUSIONS

MAH is a frequent complication of advanced cancer whether or not involving the bone. This is due to the production of cancer cells of PTHrP or, less frequently, other agents which increase plasmatic levels of calcium with several clinical consequences that may be fatal if untreated.

Currently, rehydration, promotion of calciuresis and the administration of bisphosphonates represent the standard approaches to MAH with high rates of clinical improvements. The treatment of the primary tumor itself is believed to be still the only measure impacting on the prognosis of these patients [33]. Agents which are able to interrupt RANKL mediated cascades activated by bone metastatic invasion and/or PTHrP, represent a new option for the treatment of MAH and results of ongoing clinical trials are awaited.

REFERENCES

[1]   Grill V, Martin TJ. Hypercalcemia of malignancy. Rev Endocr Metab Disord 2000; 1: 253-263.
[2]   Stewart, AF. Hypercalcemia associated with cancer. N Engl J Med 2005, 352: 373-379.
[3]   Lumachi F, Brunello A, Roma A, Basso U. Medical treatment of malignancy-associated hypercalcemia. Curr Med Chem. 2008; 15: 415-421.
[4]   Tucci M, Mosca A, Lamannaq G, *et al.* Prognostic significance of disordered calcium metabolism in hormone-refractory prostate cancer patients with metastatic bone disease. Prostate Cancer Prostatic Dis 2009; 12: 94-99.
[5]   Suva LJ, Winslow GA, Wettenhall RE, *et al.* A parathyroid hormone-related protein implicated in malignant hypercalcemia: cloning and expression. Science 1987; 237: 893-896.
[6]   Syed MA, Horwitz MJ, Tedesco MB, Garcia-Ocaña A, Wisniewski SR, Stewart AF. Parathyroid hormone-related protein-(PTHrp) stimulates renal tubular calcium reabsorption in normal human volunteers: implications for the pathogenesis of humoral hypercalcemia of malignancy. J Clin Endocrinol Metab 2001; 86: 1525-1531.

[7]   Morony S, Warmington K, Adamu S, *et al*. The inhibition of RANKL causes a greater suppression of bone resorption and hypercalcemia compared with bisphosphonates in two models of humoral hypercalcemia in malignancy. Endocrinology 2005; 146: 3235-3243.

[8]   Shivnani SB, Shelton JM, Richardson JA, Maalouf NM. Hypercalcemia of malignancy with simultaneous elevation in serum parathyroid hormone-related peptide and 1,25-dihydroxyvitamin D in a patient with metastatic renal cell carcinoma. Endocr Pract 2009; 15: 234-239.

[9]   Tanaka S, Nakamura K, Takahasi N, Suda T. Role of RANKL in physiological and pathological bone resorption and therapeutics targeting the RANKL-RANK signalling system. Immun Rev 2005; 208: 30-49.

[10]   Tanaka S, Nakamura I, Inoue J, Oda H, Nakamura K. Signal transduction pathways regulating osteoclast differentiation and function. J Bone Miner Metab 2003; 21, 123-133.

[11]   Grill V, Rankin W, Martin TJ. Parathyroid hormone-related protein (PTHrP) and hypercalcaemia. Eur J Cancer 1998; 34: 222-229.

[12]   Walji N, Chan AK, Peake DR. Common acute oncological emergencies: diagnosis, investigations and management. Postgrad Med J 2008; 84: 418-27.

[13]   Ralston SH, Coleman R, Fraser WD, *et al*. Medical management of hypercalcemia. Calcif Tissue Int 2004; 74: 1-11.

[14]   Lumachi F, Tregnaghi A, Zucchetta P, *et al*. Technetium-99m sestamibi scintigraphy and helical CT together in patients with primary hyperparathyroidism: a prospective clinical study. Br J Radiol 2004; 77: 100-103.

[15]   Lumachi F, Basso SM, Basso U. Parathyroid cancer: etiology, clinical presentation and treatment. Anticancer Res 2006; 26: 4803-4807.

[16]   Fritchie K, Zedek D, Grenache DG. The clinical utility of parathyroid hormone-related peptide in the assessment of hypercalcemia. Clin Chim Acta 2009; 402: 146-149.

[17]   Kovacs CS, MacDonald SM, Chik CL, Bruera E. Hypercalcemia of malignancy in the palliative care patient: a treatment strategy. J Pain Symptom Manage 1995; 10: 224-32.

[18]   Russel RG, Croucher PI, Rogers MJ. Bisphosphonates: pharmacology, mechanism of action and clinical uses. Osteoporos Int 9 (suppl 2): S66-S80.

[19]   Body JJ, Dumon C. Treatment of tumour-induced hypercalcaemia with the bisphosphonate pamidronate: dose-response relationship and influence of tumour type. Ann Oncol 1994; 5: 359-363.

[20]   Vinholes J, Guo CY, Purohit OP, Eastell R, Coleman RE. Evaluation of new bone resorption markers in a randomized comparison of pamidronate or clodronate for hypercalcemia of malignancy. J Clin Oncol 1997; 15: 131-138.

[21]   Thürlimann B, Waldburger R, Senn HJ, Thébaud D. Plicamycin and pamidronate in symptomatic tumor-related hypercalcemia: a prospective randomized crossover trial. Ann Oncol 2003; 14: 1468-1476.

[22]   Body JJ. Bisphosphonates for malignancy-related bone disease: current status, future developments. Support Care Cancer 2006; 14: 408-418.

[23]   Pecherstorfer M, Streunhauer EU, Rizzoli R, Wetterwald M, Berström B. Efficacy and safety of ibandronate in the treatment of hypercalcemia of malignancy: a randomized multicentric comparison to pamidronate. Support Care Cancer 2003; 11: 539-547.

[24]   Fleisch H. Bisphosphonates: mechanism of action. Endocr Rev 1998; 19: 80-100.

[25]   Bekker PJ, Holloway DL, Rasmussen AS, *et al*. a single-dose placebo-controlled study of AMG 162, a fully human monoclonal antibody to RANKL, in postmenopausal women. J Bone Min Res 2004; 19: 1059-1066.

[26]   McClung MR, Lewiecki EM, Cohen SB, *et al*. Denosumab in postmenopausal women with low bone mineral density. N Engl J Med 2006; 354: 821-31.

[27]   Body JJ, Facon T, Coleman RE, *et al*. A study of the biological receptor activator of nuclear factor-kappaB ligand inhibitor, denosumab, in patients with multiple myeloma or bone metastases from breast cancer. Clin Cancer Res 2006; 12: 1221-1228.

[28]   Body JJ, Lipton A, Gralow J, *et al*. Effects of denosumab in patients with bone metastases, with and without previous bisphosphonate exposure. J Bone Miner Res 2009, Epub. PMID: 19653815.

[29]   Sato K, Onuma E, Yocum RC, Ogata E. Treatment of malignancy-associated hypercalcemia and cachexia with humanized anti-parathyroid hormone-related protein antibody. Semin Oncol 2003; 30: 167-173.

[30]   Onuma E, Azuma Y, Saito H, *et al*. Increased renal calcium reabsorption by parathyroid hormone-related protein is a causative factor in the development of humoral hypercalcemia of malignancy refractory to osteoclastic bone resorption inhibitors. Clin Cancer Res 2005; 11: 4198-4203.

[31] Pecherstorfer M, Schilling T, Blind E, *et al*. Parathyroid hormone-related protein and life expectancy in hypercalcemia cancer patients. J Clin Endocrinol Metab 1994; 78: 1268-1270.

[32] Hudes G, Carducci M, Tomczak P, et al. Temsirolimus, interferon alpha, or both for advanced renal-cell carcinoma. N Engl J Med 2007; 356: 2271-2281.

[33] Lumachi F, Brunello A, Roma A, Basso U. Cancer-induced hypercalcemia. Anticancer Res 2009; 29: 1551-1556.

CHAPTER 4

Acute Hypercalcemia

Fabiana Nascimben

Emergency Department, S. Maria degli Angeli Hospital, 33170 Pordenone, Italy

Abstract: Hypercalcemia is a frequent condition, especially in cancer patients, sometimes difficult to diagnose because of its clinical presentation, mimicking other diseases. Severe elevation of serum calcium generally gives mild and non-specific symptoms, ranging from fatigue, nausea, vomiting, abdominal pain, and up to mental status deterioration and cardiac arrhythmias. It is crucial to recognize acute hypercalcemia soon, and treat it aggressively. The severity of clinical findings depends on both the calcium level and the rate at which it develops. The first line treatment is massive rehydration with intravenous saline 0.9% to reach normovolemia, using invasive or non-invasive monitoring. This helps eliminating calcium excretion in the urine. When hemodynamic status or renal function is impaired, dialysis should be considered. Only when normovolemic status is achieved and renal function restored, furosemide administration can help to further increase urinary excretion of calcium. The second step is to inhibit osteoclastic bone resorption, which is possible with both bisphosphonate and non-bisphosphonate drugs. After the emergency treatment, it is important to diagnose and treat the underlying disease, such as hematological malignancy or other malignancies, while patients with primary hyperparathyroidism should be considered for surgery within a few days.

INTRODUCTION

One of the most challenging experiences in the Emergency Department is looking forward to discovering diseases that at first are not what they seem to be. Disorders of serum calcium concentration generally gives mild and non specific symptoms, including fatigue, anorexia, depression, vomiting, constipations, weakness, abdominal pain, and ECG modification. Severe hypercalcemia can also cause acute pancreatitis and peptic ulcer. So it is important to think about calcium level when a patient "looks bad" or has mild clinical findings.

Ninety-nine percent of calcium is inside the bone, about 1% extracellular, and 0.1% intracellular. Its metabolism and regulation are complex, and the range of its circulating concentration is narrow, rising from 9 to 10 mg/dL (2.25-2.50 mmol/L). Calcium levels are usually measured as mg/dL, which can be converted into mmol/L by dividing by 4, or in mEq/L by dividing by 2 (see Chapter 5).

The calcium regulation depends on calcitonin, parathyroid hormone (PTH), vitamin D, phosphate, albumin level, pH, and calcium itself. We consider hypercalcemia when calcium value rises over 2.55-2.62 mmol/L, but it is extremely important to consider the ionized amount. Calcemia means the overall amount of this cation, but in the human body calcium is about 40% bound to proteins, especially albumin, 10% bound to organic anions, and is 50% ionized. Table **1** reports the classification of hypercalcemia (see also Chapter 5).

Table 1: Classification of hypercalcemia.

	Normal value	Mild	Moderate	Severe	Life-threatening
mmol/L	2.15-2.60	2.6-3.0	3.1-3.5	> 3.5	> 4
mg/dL	8.5-10.3	10.5-12.0	12.1-14.0	> 14.0	> 15-16

Growth or decrease in albumin level can modify the ionized part, the only biologically active [1]. With normal levels of albumin (4 gr/dL) and normal pH (7. 4) the ionized calcium in adults is 1.13-1.32

mmol/L (4.6-5.3 mg/dL). Normal values of total calcemia are commonly considered between 2.15 and 2.6 mmol/L (8.5-10.5 mg/dL). We consider hypercalcemia when calcium levels rise 2.6 mmol/L. Remember: 1 mg/dL of albumin binds 0.2 mmol/L (0.8 mg/dL) of calcium. The next formula can help to "adjust" serum total calcium according to albuminemia:

Adjusted calcium (mmol/L) = serum total calcium (mmol/L) + (0.025 × albumin g/L)

Also, the pH value can modify calcium levels, changing its affinity to proteins: alkalosis improves calcium affinity to proteins, diminishing the ionized part, while acidosis decreases affinity to proteins, and increases ionized calcium. If pH decrease to 0.1, ionized calcium rises to 0.05 mmol/L. The following formula k is 0.05 (mmol/L) or 0.2 (mg/dL) helps correcting calcium compared to pH:

Calcium corrected for pH = total calcium + [k × (7.4 – pH)]

CLINICAL FINDINGS

In the Emergency Department hypercalcemia is the most frequent neoplastic-related disorder, and can be life-threatening [2]. Although, many conditions can cause hypercalcemia, primary hyperparathyroidism is the most common cause followed by malignancy associated hypercalcemia (MAH), in which other tissues can produce proteins that mimic the parathyroid hormone (see Chapter 3). Drug-related syndromes, and granulomatous diseases, such as sarcoidosis, tuberculosis, and Wegener's disease, are other causes of hypercalcemia [3] (Fig. 1).

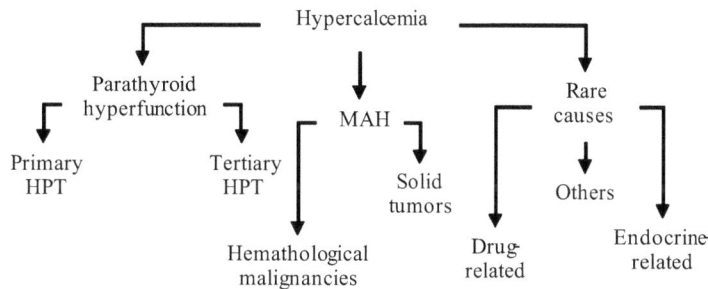

Figure 1: Main causes of hypercalcemia. HPT = hyperparathyroidism, MAH = malignancy-associated hypercalcemia.

The severity of hypercalcemia depends on both serum calcium levels and the rate at which it develops: lesser the time, more the toxicity. Remember that MAH can evolve dramatically when there is concomitant dehydration, volume depletion and renal impairment. In patients with acute hypercalcemia the goal is, first of all, to recognize the problem.

Hypercalcemic patients can present a broad spectrum of symptoms, most of all mild and non-specific, rising from non-specific weakness till mental status alteration (i.e. lethargy, depression, and stupor), as well as cardiac arrhythmias.

Frequently, patients exhibit signs of renal function impairment, such as polyuria due to a reduction in urinary concentration capacity (nephogenic diabetes insipidus), volume depletion, and an increase in the serum creatinine levels.

Gastrointestinal impairments, like nausea, vomiting, abdominal pain, and constipation, can be also observed. When the calcium levels are high for a long time, peptic ulcers and acute pancreatitis may occur.

Rare but serious cases of skin ulcers and necrosis are reported, related to parathyroid adenoma, probably due to calciphylaxis [4]. Another rare clinical feature is loss of vision due to the band keratopathy, a horizontal band across the cornea due to subepithelial calcium phosphate deposits [1, 5]. In patients with severe (>3.5 mmol/L) hypercalcemia, cognitive alteration, mental confusion, hyporeflexia, stupor and coma may be observed [6].

Looking at the Electrocardiogram (ECG), there are some typical alterations: shortening of QT interval (hypercalcemia directly shortens the myocardial potential), increasing of PR interval, and more rarely Osborn wave, especially with concomitant hypothermia [7]. Symptoms mimicking acute myocardial infarction with ST elevation, but normal angiography and normalization of ECG with normalization of calcium levels, have been reported [8].

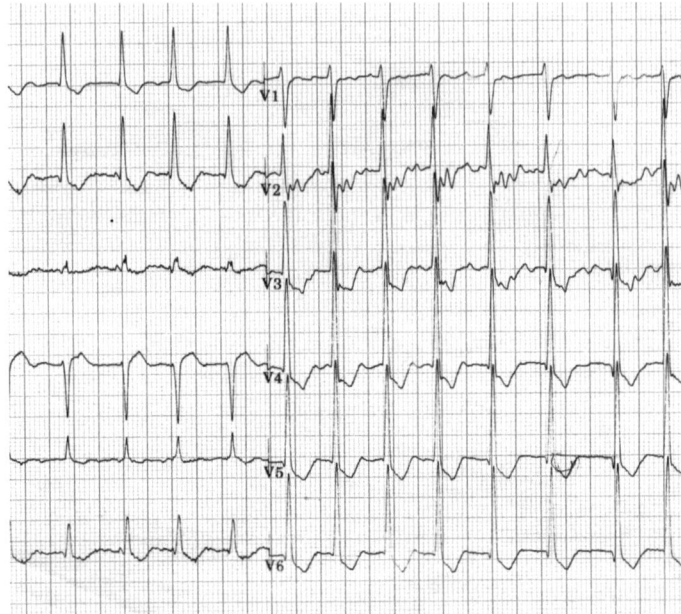

Figure 2: Electrocardiogram demonstrating atrial fibrillation with ST alterations, in a 76-year-old woman admitted in the Emergency Department with stupor. Laboratory data showed severe hypercalcemia (4.2 mmol/L), and no troponine elevation. Na^+ and K^+ were normal, while parathyroid hormone serum level was 252 pg/mL (reference range 12-72). Neck ultrasonography showed a parathyroid adenoma of the left inferior parathyroid gland sized 35 mm. In spite of the emergency treatment (hydration with saline and loop diuretics, intraperitoneal dialysis) and parathyroidectomy, the patient died of ventricular fibrillation and cardiac arrest.

TREATMENT

In the Emergency Department, it is important to assess the gravity of the patient. First of all, consider the ABC assessment: Airway-Breathing-Circulation. It is important to evaluate and preserve the vital functions. If indicated, start with Advanced Cardiac Life Support (ACLS), following guidelines [9].

If the patient does not need resuscitation, check neurological status, arterial blood pressure, cardiac pulses, oxygen saturation and temperature. Then, assess at least an intravenous access, take blood samples for blood cell count, glucose, renal and liver function index, pancreatic enzymes, Na^+, K^+ and calcium levels, creatine phosphokinase (CPK), troponin, and hemogasanalysis. Finally, perform an ECG in 12 leads, and place a urine catheter with urometer.

Because of both dehydration and hypercalcemia, a huge amount of fluids could be necessary. Consider central vein catheterization, that gives the advantage of measuring central vein pressure (CVP), and having a good vascular access.

Treatment should be initiated for all patients with symptoms and in patients with moderate or severe hypercalcemia (>3 mmol/L) even if minimally symptomatic.

The following severity index and admission criteria should be considered:

- Severe dehydration
- Mental status alteration
- Renal impairment
- Cardiac arrhythmias
- Ionized calcium level
- Paralytic ileum
- Nausea or vomiting
- Low social level

There are five keystones of therapy:

i) Restore normovolemia to prevent renal impairment

ii) Restore renal function and enhance renal excretion of calcium

iii) Dialysis

iv) Inhibit osteoclastic bone resorption

v) Reduce intestinal calcium absorption

During the emergency treatment, check and monitor vital signs, diuresis and mental status every hour. Calcium, magnesium, renal electrolytes, and pH should be tested every 6-12 hours, and corrected when needed.

Restore Normovolemia

Generally, the patient needs a lot of fluids because there is an osmotic urination due to calciuresis, leading to diabetes insipidus. The first approach is to restore normovolemia. Give saline 0.9%, 200-500 mL/h in the first hours, followed by 100-200 mL/h for 24/h, monitoring CVP, blood pressure, cardiac and renal function, and mental status. Try to maintain diuresis around 100-150 mL/h. The aim of rehydration is to restore a normovolemic status and promote urinary calcium excretion, reducing hypercalcemia.

Restore Renal Function and Enhance Renal Excretion of Calcium

In patients without CVP increment and/or without heart failure, once the hydration state has been assessed and renal function restored, only rehydration could be enough for increasing calcium elimination.

Euvolemic status is acheived, when diuresis is at least 100 mL/h. only in patients with labile hemodynamic compensation, a diuretic loop is obtained, like furosemide, 20-40 mg intravenously 2-4 times/day, together with saline. Furosemide can worsen renal impairment and can provoke hypokalemia. Thiazide diuretics are contraindicated because they promote intra-tubular reabsorption of calcium that increases serum calcium levels.

Dialysis

Dialysis is indicated in case of severe hypercalcemia with mental status impairment and heart failure or renal insufficiency, when massive hydration is contraindicated.

The effect is observed in a few hours and lasts up to 2-3 days. The peritoneal dialysis has the same effect as hemodialysis, but it takes longer. By changing dialysis fluids composition you can add phosphorus and compensate hypophosphoremia.

Inhibit Osteoclastic Bone Resorption

There are many drugs that inhibit osteoclastic bone resorption by different mechanisms. The choice depends on the severity of hypercalcemia, allergies, other drugs used, and renal function. Some old drugs are over, but they can be of choice in selected patients, for a second-line therapy. Two main groups of drugs should be considered: bisphosphonates and non-bisphosphonates drugs (Fig. **3**).

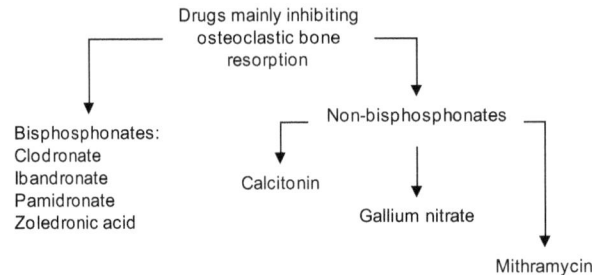

Figure 3: Drugs inhibiting osteoclastic bone resorption and/or osteoblastic bone forming.

In case of acute MAH or another severe hypercalcemic status, bisphosphonates are safe drugs. Currently, bisphosphonates are the drugs of choice in most of the patients after correct hydration, but they take 2-4 days before acting, and their effect lasts up to 4 weeks. The mechanism of action is both inhibiting osteoclasts activity (bone resorption) and stimulating osteoblastic bone forming. Usually, intravenous administration is the treatment of choice, while for maintenance there are oral formulations, not useful in the emergency setting [10].

Clodronate is now less used for its gastrointestinal toxicity, and because other bisphosphonates are more effective.

Ibandronate is available in intravenous and oral formulations. For acute hypercalcemia the dose is 6 mg of infusion over 1 hour, every 3-4 weeks: the effect starts 24 hours later, and the nadir is on the fifth day. Being that in some trials it showed that less renal impairment could be the drug of choice in patients with mild renal impairment, or in patients receiving other nephrotoxic drugs [11].

Pamidronate is a second generation drug. It is indicated for the treatment of moderate or severe hypercalcemia in patients with MAH, with or without bone metastases. Pamidronate is eliminated by the kidney. Due to the risk of significant impairment of urinary concentrating ability, single dose of pamidronate disodium should not exceed 90 mg, and the duration of infusion should be no less than 2 hours. The effectiveness starts in 2 days, and the calcium nadir is expected in 6-7 days. If serum calcium ranges between 2.7 and 3.5 mmol/L: give 60 mg in 250-500 0.9% saline or 5% glucose solution over 2-4 hours. If serum calcium is > 3.5 mmol/L: give 90 mg in 500 ml isotonic solution or 5% glucose solution over 4 hours. Check serum calcium for 6-7 days, for the risk of hypocalcemia. Be aware of Renal impairment decreases in calcium phosphorus and magnesium. A Rare collateral effect could be osteonecrosis of the jaw. Do not Use pamidronate in pregnant women.

Zoledronic acid is a third generation drug, mainly indicated for patients with MAH. It is safe and effective, 10,000 times more potent than etidronate, with short infusion. Dose: 4 mg in 100 mL 0.9% saline or 5% glucose solution in at least 15 minutes. No dose correction is necessary if creatinine clearance is > 40 mL/h. The effect starts in 2 days and lasts up to 4 weeks. Be aware of an increasing effect with Concomitant infusion of aminoglycosides.

Calcitonin is a polypeptide hormone physiologically produced by the C cells in the thyroid gland, which acts directly on both osteoclasts and renal cells, via specific receptors on the cell surface. It is more expensive and can cause severe allergic reactions in respect of bisphosphonates. Nevertheless, calcitonin is useful in severe hypercalcemia, when rapid effect is needed and dialysis is not immediately available. Indications are neurological impairment with severe or life-threatening hypercalcemia (> 4 mmol/L), and no response to aggressive rehydration or dialysis is not available. The usual dose is 100 UI of salmon derived calcitonin every 6-8 hours. In extremely severe and selected cases, 5-10 UI/kg in 500 ml 0.9%, saline solution over 6 hours can be used. Calcitonin can be used together with bisphosphonates infusion, and it should be the drug of choice for patients with renal failure unable to receive pamidronate or zoledronic acid, or when ibandronate is not available. Be aware of tachyphylaxis that can occur after 2-3 days. The effect starts in 6-12 hours and lasts for 2-3 days.

Gallium nitrate is a non-cytotoxic anticancer drug, more effective than calcitonin or bisphosphonates. It may work by directly inhibiting osteoclasts, reducing tubular reabsorption and solubilization of hydroxyapatite crystals. Today the indications are limited for the treatment of patients refractory to bisphosphonates. The common dosage is 100-200 mg/m^2 in continuous infusion over 5 days. The effect arises in 5 days and goes on 7-10 days.

Mithramycin is an osteoclast's RNA inhibitor, less effective compared to pamidronate, useful in association with bisphosphonates. Dose: 25 µg/kg in 5% glucose solution in 4-6 hrs every 24-48 hrs for 7 days maximum. Effect expected in 12 hrs, lasts up to 2-4 days. Contraindications are renal and liver impairment, chemotherapy and hemorrhagic conditions.

Reduce Intestinal Calcium Absorption

Glucocorticoids reduce intestinal calcium absorption and renal excretion. They also reduce malignant cells. Their effectiveness is proven in hematological conditions (multiple myeloma, leukemia), sarcoidosis, and vitamin A & D intoxication, representing the first-line of treatment. Usually, they are not effective in primary hyperparathyroidism. The main drugs available are prednisone (20-50 mg orally, 2 times a day), and hydrocortisone (200-400 mg daily for 3-5 days). The effectiveness is expected in 2-3 days, lasting for 1-2 weeks. Be aware of hyperglycemia.

A decisional algorithm is showed in Fig. **4**.

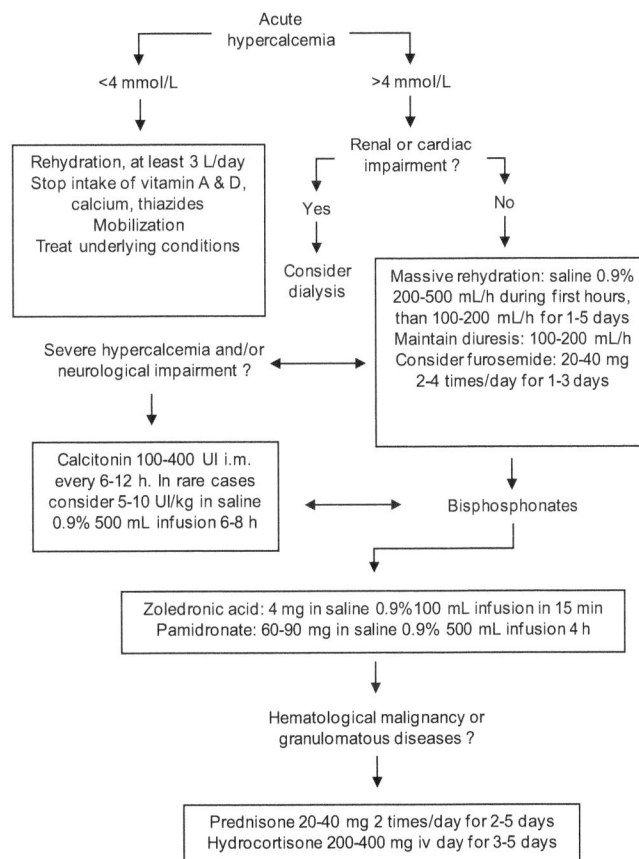

Figure 4: Suggested decisional algorithm in patients with acute hypercalcemia.

CONCLUSIONS

For the Emergency Room physician, it is important to recognize the disease and promptly treat it, according to the evidence-based medicine.

Now, the first line treatment is massive rehydration if possible, or dialysis in patients with hemodynamic or renal impairment. Almost immediately bisphosphonate drugs can be started. The patient needs to be admitted in a monitored Care Unit for aggressive treatment, at least during the first 24 hours, or more if needed. At the same time, a diagnostic plan to recognize the underlying disease should be started in order to focus on the appropriate treatment.

REFERENCES

[1]   Assadi F. Hypercalcemia: an evidence-based approach to clinical cases. Iran J Kidney Dis 2009; 3: 71-79.
[2]   Lumachi F, Brunello A, Roma A, Basso U. Medical treatment of malignancy-associated Hypercalcemia. Curr Med Chem 2008; 15: 415-421.
[3]   Sato T, Tsuru T, Hagiwara K, *et al.* Sarcoidosis with acute recurent polyarthritis and hypercalcemia. Intern Med 2006; 45: 363-368.
[4]   Joukhadar R, Bright T. Calciphylaxis in primary hyperparathyroidism: a case report and brief review. South Med J 2009; 102: 318-321.
[5]   Wilson KS, Alexander S, Chisholm IA. Band keratopathy in hypercalcemia of myeloma. Can Med Assoc J 1982; 126: 1324-1315.
[6]   Weiss-Guillet EM, Takala J, Jacob SM. Diagnosis and management of electrolyte emergencies. Best Pract Res Clin Endocrinol Metab 2003;17: 623-651.
[7]   Diercks DB, Shumaik GM, Harrigan RA, Brady WJ, Chan TC. Electrocardiographic manifestations: electrolyte abnormalities. J Emerg Med 2004; 27: 153-160.
[8]   Nishi SP, Barbagelata NA, Atar S, Birnbaum Y, Tuero E. Hypercalcemia-induced ST-segment elevation mimicking acute myocardial infarction. J Electrocardiol 2006; 39: 298-300.
[9]   ECC Committee, Subcommittees and Task Forces of the American Heart Association. 2005 American Heart Association Guidelines for Cardiopulmonary Resuscitation and Emergency Cardiovascular Care. Circulation 2005; 112: IV1-IV203.
[10]   Fraser WD. Hyperparathyroidism. Lancet 2009; 374: 145-158.
[11]   Lumachi F, Brunello A, Roma A, Basso U. Cancer-induced hypercalcemia. Anticancer Res 2009; 29: 1551-1556.

CHAPTER 5

Laboratory & Hypercalcemia

Piero Cappelletti[1] and Renato Tozzoli[2]

[1]*Department of Clinical Pathology, S. Maria degli Angeli Hospital, 33170 Pordenone, Italy and* [2]*Department of Clinical Chemistry & Microbiology, City Hospital, 33053 Latisana, Italy*

Abstract: Hypercalcemia, defined as serum total calcium "adjusted" for the serum albumin concentration above the upper limit of the population reference interval, can develop either in a context of a known disease (renal failure, malignancy, or endocrine diseases) or an unexpected result in a routine biochemical testing. The first step is confirming that it is "true" hypercalcemia, excluding pre-analytical, biological, and analytical interferences. A serum calcium value >2.65-2.70 mmol/L (10.8 mg/dL) is very unlikely to be due to analytic variations. However, only ionized calcium correctly assesses the calcium balance and should be the test of choice. In the diagnostic algorithm, which requires assessment of renal function by serum creatinine or estimated glomerular fraction rate, the key step is the determination of intact parathyroid hormone (PTH), together with 25-hydroxyvitamin D [25(OH)]D, for differential diagnosis between PTH-mediated and non-PTH-mediated hypercalcemia. In primary hyperparathyroidism, laboratory findings related to calcium balance and renal function, together with bone mineral density, are important guideline elements in patients with symptomatic primary HPT. In those undergoing parathyroidectomy, the intraoperative measurement of PTH by a quick assay may predict operative outcome. In familial hyperparathyroidism, genetic sequencing can provide useful information and it is necessary for a definitive diagnosis, and adequate management of relatives. In severe malignancy-associated hypercalcemia, calcium-phosphate balance and renal function tests are useful for monitoring the course of disease, and the effects of medical therapy. In differential diagnosis with granulomatous disorders, 25(OH)D measurement is suggested, while PTH-related protein assay is not recommended as a routine test.

INTRODUCTION

Calcium is essential to homeostasis and functioning of multiple organ systems. Its circulating concentration is maintained within a very tight physiologic range: between 2.25 and 2.50 mmol/L (9-10 mg/dL). The concentration of calcium in SI units (mmol/L) is obtained multiplying concentration in mg/dL × 0.25. About 50-60% of blood calcium is bound to plasma proteins, mostly albumin, or forms a complex with phosphate or citrate, while the rest is the ionized form, also termed as "active", "circulating" or "free" calcium (Fig. **1**).

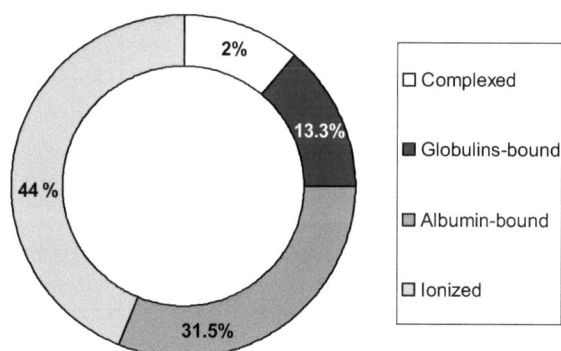

Figure 1: Forms of calcium in the blood.

Under physiological conditions, the *ionized calcium* (iCa) concentration is regulated by parathyroid hormone (PTH), calcitonin, and 1, 25-dihydroxyvitamin D [1,25(OH)$_2$D] through mutual interactions on target organs such as kidney, bone and intestine (see Chapter 1). This tight minute-to-minute control is mainly based on the parathyroid chief cells, which are the most important calcium-sensing cells in the body, although both chief cells and oxyphil parathyroid cells are associated with secretory functions. The inverse sigmoidal relationship between PTH secretion and iCa concentration means that very small changes in the latter lead to immediate physiologic responses that restore the concentration to normal. A decrease in iCa of only 0.03 mmol/L results in a doubling of PTH secretion.

The key role in this delicate homeostatic system depends on the extracellular calcium-sensing receptor (CaSR), whose affinity for iCa is within the millimolar range.

The set-point of CaSR, defined as the extracellular calcium concentration causing half-maximum inhibition of PTH secretion, is 1.1-1.3 mmol/L, which corresponds to the reference values of plasma iCa levels. The reference range of total serum calcium (tCa) concentrations in the blood varies slightly with age, being higher during bone growth (Table **1**).

Table 1: Reference range for calcium, according to age.

Total Calcium	mmol/L	mg/dL
Child	2.20-2.68	8.8-10.7
Adult	2.10-2.55	8.4-10.2
Ionized calcium		
At birth	1.30-1.60	5.2-6.4
Neonate	1.20-1.48	4.8-5.9
Child	1.20-1.38	4.8-5.5
Adult	1.16-1.32	4.6-5.3

Hypercalcemia is usually defined as serum total calcium, "adjusted" for the serum albumin concentration above the upper limit of the population reference interval. Different ranges of upper limits (2.55-2.62 mmol/L) are reported, depending on method and population studies. A threshold of 2.65 mmol/L at the upper end of adult ranges is suggested to trigger investigation, while 1.35 mmol/L means a decision limit for iCa to define a hypercalcemia [1]. Although there are no formal guidelines, hypercalcemia can be classified as mild, moderate and severe (Table **2**). Some authors quote different thresholds (i.e. 2.88 mmol/L as mild *vs.* moderate, 3.40 mmol/L as moderate *vs.* severe).

Table 2: Classification of hypercalcemia. Adapted from [2].

Mild	< 3.0 mmol/L (12 mg/dL)
Moderate	>3.0 mmol/L (12 mg/dL) <3.5 mmol/L (14 mg/dL)
Severe	>3.5 mmol/L (14 mg/dL)

DIAGNOSING HYPERCALCEMIA

What does "true" hypercalcemia mean ? To evaluate hypercalcemia, particularly mild hypercalcemia, it is important to rule out pseudohypercalcemia ("factitious" hypercalcemia), excluding biological, pre-analytical, and analytic influencing factors. About 50% of tCa is present as iCa, 40% is protein-bound, and 10% is complexed with citrate and phosphate. Because elevated concentrations of plasma proteins may increase tCa levels, it is recommended to "adjust" serum tCa value at least for its main influencing factor, serum albumin (Alb), by appropriate formulas (Table **3**).

Table 3: Relationship between calcium and albumin concentrations ([1]Landeson JH *et al.* J Clin Endocrinol Metab 1978; 48: 393-387. [2]Pedersen KO. Scand J Clin Lab Invest 1978; 38: 659-667. [3]Clase CM *et al.* Nephrol Dial Transplant 2000; 15: 1841-1846).

Adjusted calcium (mmol/L) = serum total calcium (mmol/L) + (0.025 × albumin g/L)[1]
Corrected calcium = serum total calcium + [0.00839 × (32.9 – albumin)][2]
Corrected calcium (mg/dL) = serum total calcium – [0.707 × (albumin – 3.4)][3]

Total calcium is lowered by 0.2 mmol/L for every 1 mg/dL of Alb or protein above normal levels and/or corrected to a normalized Alb of 40 g/L. Nevertheless, the adjustment is an approximation, that may be inaccurate particularly at extreme Alb concentrations, which depends on the upper limit of the reference range, analytical imprecision, and method differences of Alb. Inter-individual differences, rare cases of analbuminemia and, in addition, marked hyperglobulinemia (i.e. monoclonal protein) can strongly increase tCa levels, without altering iCa levels. Thus, "active" iCa cannot be accurately calculated from tCa. Measuring iCa, tCa, and total CO_2 (tCO_2) in mmol/L, and Alb is in g/L, the best predictive formula for iCa calculation is the following [3]:

$$iCa = 0.5\ tCa - 0.005\ Alb - 0.002\ tCO_2 + 0.2934$$

Pseudohypercalcemia can occur also for pre-analytical causes, when albumin is concentrated in a blood sample secondary to dehydration or prolonged tourniquet placement. Venous stasis (between 1 and 3 minutes after application) could produce changes of 0.12-0.25 mmol/L in tCa and 2-3% in iCa, because hemoconcentration causes hyperproteinemia, and localized lactate and acid production alters the ratio of calcium bound/unbound to proteins. Although there is no general agreement to these data, the advice that the tourniquet application should be brief (<1 minute) before a specimen is collected, seems reasonable [4]. Fig. **2** shows the diagnostic algorithm for hypercalcemia.

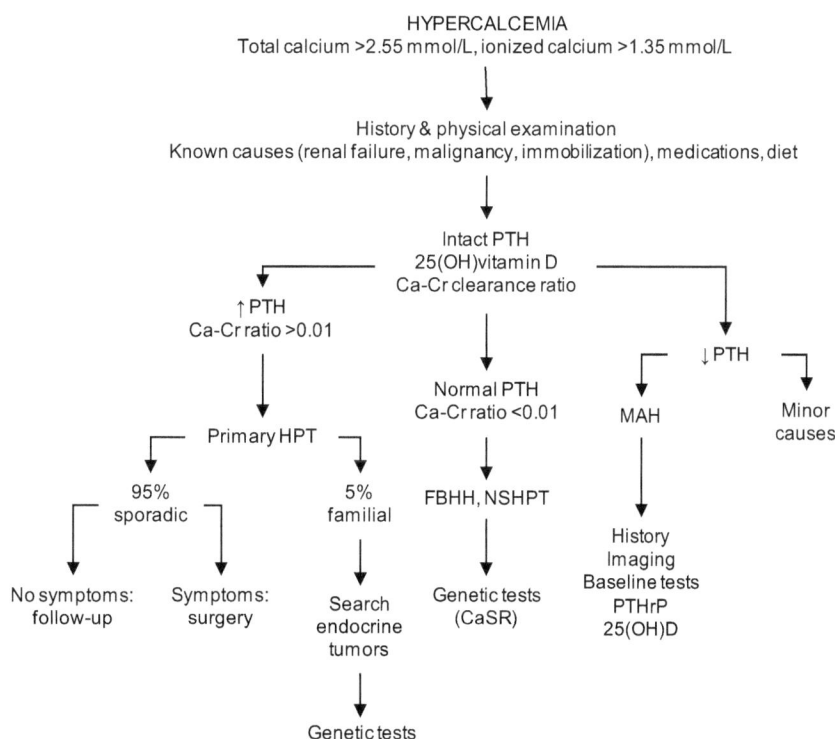

Figure 2: Diagnostic algorithm for hypercalcemia. HPT = hyperparathyroidism, FBHH = familial benign hypocalciuric hypocalcemia, NSHPT = neonatal severe hyperparathyroidism.

Other pre-analytical sources of error in tCa determination may be hemolysis, a well known interfering factor in clinical chemistry methods and non-fasting state, while a high concentration of fatty acid underestimates tCa. From the analytical point of view, some authors [5] stress that the desirable imprecision for calcium based on biological variation is narrow (0.9%), much less than the mandatory goal (±1 mg/dL) of Accreditation Bodies (i.e. CLIA). However, values more than 3 standard deviations outside the population mean (approximately 2.7 mmol/L) are statistically very unlikely to be related to analytical variations. Thus, many authors recommend confirming hypercalcemia by repeated (two or three) measurements, while others suggest the iCa measurement [1, 6].

The 2002 workshop on asymptomatic primary hyperparathyroidism (WAPHPT) guidelines [7], did not recommend routine testing of iCa in patients with mild hypercalcemia, because most physicians do not have access to a facility that can produce an accurate measurement. Therefore, tCa is still being measured for diagnostic purpose of hypercalcemia, despite its limitations. However, iCa must be measured to accurately make a diagnosis of calcium imbalance determining "true" hypercalcemia. In most patients with multiple myeloma and severe bone destruction, as well in those with malignancy-associated hypercalcemia (MAH), tCa is elevated without an increase of iCa (see Chapter 3). On the other hand, iCa is more sensitive in diagnosing asymptomatic primary hyperparathyroidism (HPT): its blood concentrations are elevated in 90-95% of patients, while tCa is elevated in 80-85% [1].

Indeed, in most clinical centers the measure of iCa is easily available for hospital and primary care physicians, despite some limits such as cost and technical issues [6]. If hypercalcemia develops in a context of a known disease (i.e. renal failure, malignancy, or endocrine diseases), the cause may be apparent. If not, the first step is a carefully performed history to eliminate some minor causes, keeping in mind the main causes of hypercalcemia, such as HPT and MAH. Setting, history and the age of patients are taken into consideration. (Table **4**).

Table 4: Anamnesis in differential diagnosis between primary hyperparathyroidism (PHPT) and malignancy-associated hypercalcemia (MAH). NSHPT = neonatal severe hyperparathyroidism.

	Setting	**Clinical features**	**Age (peak)**
PHPT			
Sporadic	Outpatients	Chronic mild hypercalcemia, routine testing unexpected result	50-60 years
Hereditary		Chronic mild hypercalcemia (except NSHPT)	20 years
MAH	Inpatients	Acute rising hypercalcemia, symptoms of underlying disease	No peak

Because of the often non-specific and insidious clinical features of hypercalcemia, the diagnosis must be confirmed and directed by further laboratory measurements. Once hypercalcemia is confirmed by iCa, the intact PTH (iPTH) assay plays a crucial role to differentiate PTH-mediated from non-PTH-mediated hypercalcemia.

The 2002 WAPHPT guidelines [7] suggest measuring the first step of the diagnostic algorithm the urinary excretion of calcium (as 24-h calciuria). Not only to rule out familial benign hypocalciuric hypercalcemia (FBHH) syndrome, but also for giving a general measure of the renal burden for handling calcium, as well as to assess the renal function by creatinine clearance (Cr-clearance). For this reason, several authors [8] indicate the ratio of calcium clearance to creatinine clearance (CaCr-clearance ratio) as a more helpful tool for differential diagnosis of FBHH. Features suggestive of FBHH are mild hypercalcemia and relative hypocalciuria, with normal PTH, or persistent hypercalciuria after an attempted parathyroidectomy (Table **5**). Definitive diagnosis requires study of the CASR gene (see below).

Table 5: Differential diagnosis between sporadic primary hyperparathyroidism (HPT), familial primary HPT, and familial benign hypocalciuric hypercalcemia (FBHH) / neonatal severe primary HPT (NSHPT). Modified from [8].

Parameters	Sporadic HHPT	Familial HPT	FBHH/NSHPT
Age (years) at diagnosis median (range)	63 (31-93)	26 (12-74)	4 (0.1-26)
Serum total calcium, mmol/L median (range)	2.78 (2.41-4.36)	2.79 (2.57-3.36)	2.91 (2.84-3.30)
Serum PTH, pg/mL median (range)	137 (69-1301)	174 (83.8-414.0)	43.5 (34.1-56)
Osteoporosis (frequency)	60.2%	66%	0%
Kidney stones (frequency)	43.1%	40%	0%

The 2008 WAPHPT guidelines [9] suggest the use of the estimated glomerular filtration ratio (eGFR) to be a more accurate test of renal function. When serum iPTH is elevated, a diagnosis of primary HPT is easily made, especially if clinical manifestations are present. Unfortunately, most patients are asymptomatic, and iPTH may be only high-normal. Because of frequent coexistence of mild hypophosphatemia (due to the PTH-induced decrease of renal threshold for phosphate clearance), and mild hypochloremic metabolic acidosis (due to PTH-induced increase in renal excretion of bicarbonate), some authors suggested to measure serum phosphate and chloride to favor the differential diagnosis between primary HPT and MAH [1].

Clinicians also use a chloride/phosphate ratio as evidence for HPT (Table **6**). However, serum phosphate may be also normal or low, especially in MAH syndrome due to parathyroid hormone-related protein (PTHrP) production, while chloride is increased in only 40% of patients. Thus, the use of those formulas is no longer suggested.

Table 6: Laboratory testing helpful in differential diagnosis between malignancy-associated hypercalcemia (MAH) and primary hyperparathyroidism (PHPT). Modified from [1].

Parameters	HPT	MAH
Calcemia	<3.13 mmol/L (<12.5 mg/dL)	>3.13 mmol/L (>12.5 mg/dL)
Intact PTH	Elevated or high-normal	Suppressed
Chloride	>103 mmol/L (>103 mEq/L)	<103 mmol/L (<103 mEq/L)
Phosphate	Normal to low	Variable
Cl/ PO_4 ratio	>102 (Cl & PO_4 mmol/L) >33 (Cl & PO_4 mg/dL)	<102 (Cl & PO_4 mmol/L) <33 (Cl & PO_4 mg/dL)
Calciuria	High	Very high

The interpretation of iPTH is now related to the quality of the technical method, and to optimal reference intervals based on coexisting 25-hydroxyvitamin D [25(OH)D] levels. In patients with primary HPT, 1,25(OH)$_2$D (calcitriol), which is under direct control of PTH, may be high or high-normal, while 25(OH)D (calcidiol), which reflects the total body vitamin store, is normal. However, because of the presence of vitamin D deficiency, it complicates the interpretation of PTH assays. The 2008 WAPHPT [9] suggests that the level of 25(OH)D should be assessed in all patients suspected of having primary HPT. The majority (95%) of cases of primary HPT are sporadic, depending on an acquired somatic chromosomal abnormality, while 5% are familial HPT and are the result of germline mutations in genes, such as CASR (also defined CaSR), hyperparathyroidism 2 (HRPT2), cyclin-dependent kinase inhibitor 1B (CDKN1B), and MEN1. Young age and clinical features suggest the diagnosis, and molecular methods for genetic analysis are necessary only for definitive assessment [8].

If iPTH is low or suppressed in the absence of consumption of vitamin D or analogues, MAH should be suspected, especially when hypercalcemia is pronounced (>3.25 mmol/L). Except rare small neuroendocrine tumors (i.e. VIPoma), solid tumors causing MAH are generally large and readily apparent, and thus PTHrP should not routinely be measured. Plasma vitamin D should be measured only when T cell lymphoma or granulomatous diseases (i.e. sarcoidosis) are included in the differential diagnosis When MAH has been excluded in hypercalciuric non-PTH mediated hypercalcemia, less common causes should be investigated.

STANDARD BIOCHEMICAL FINDINGS

Total calcium is usually measured by spectrophotometric dye binding assay (i.e. arsenazo III, o-cresophtalein complexone), or by ion-selective electrodes (ISE) after releasing calcium into the free state by the addition of acid [10].

Proper collection is very important to avoid pre-analytical and analytical sources of error. Hyperlipidemia from non-fasting patients, hemoconcentration, hemolysis from incorrect venipuncture, posture modification, and physical exercise (15-20 minutes) before phlebotomy determine an increase of 4-7% in calcium levels [11] (Table **7**).

Table 7: Pre-analytic interferences in some tests for diagnosing hypercalcemia. *Patients often do not collect urine excreted in 24 hours with precision.

Parameters	Patient	Collection	Conservation
Calcemia (tCa)	Albumin concentration Hyperglobulinemia Fasting	Venous stasis Posture Exercise	
Calciuria (uCa)	Calcium diet	24-h collection*	Acidified urine
Ionized calcium (iCa)	Hyperventilation	Anaerobic sample Heparin effect	Analysis <1 h
Phosphate	Fasting	Hemolysis	Centrifugation < 1 h
Creatinine-clearance		24-h collection*	

Desirable analytical specifications were defined on the basis of biological variation: analytical variation (CVa) 1.0%, desirable bias (B) 0.8% [12]. Unfortunately, the methods in use do not always reach the proposed goals of analytic performance (Table **8**).

Table 8: Desirable and actual analytic performances of some tests for diagnosing hypercalcemia. * From [5] **Mean of different analytic methods.

	Desirable analytic performances based on biological variation*		Actual analytic performances at decision limit**	
	CVa%	Bias %	CV%	Bias%
s Calcium	1.0	0.8	1.5	2.0
u Calcium	13.8	11.5	3.5	5.1
Ionized Calcium	0.9	0.7	0.9	-0.02
s Phosphate	4.3	3.2	1.3	-2.8
u Phosphate	13.2	9.4	1.7	-2.8
s Creatinine	2.7	3.8	1.7	-0.3
u Creatinine	12.0	8.6	3.8	-3.0
s BAP	3.1	9.0	3.6	7.1
s C-Telopeptide	4.8	8.0	6.9	4
s Pancreatic amylase	5.9	8.0	2.5	-11.0

Interpretation of serum tCa levels depends on individual characteristics of patients, as well as pre-analytical and analytical influencial factors. Patients with primary HPT usually have chronic mild-to-high calcium levels, but in 10-20% of cases they have concentrations in the high end of reference range [11]. Mild hypercalcemia is also present in up to 10-20% of patients treated with lithium for bipolar disorders, in 7-8% of those treated with thiazide diuretics, and in patients with prolonged immobilization (>1 week, peak at 10 weeks), or during the recovery phase of rhabdomyolysis. Very high (>3.5 mmol/L) levels of tCa, and a rapid increase of hypercalcemia usually suggest a MAH syndrome [13].

The usefulness of reference range for diagnosing individual patient and the critical difference for correct monitoring of patients are shown in Table **9**.

Table 9: Biological interpretation of some tests for diagnosing hypercalcemia. * From [5] ** Modified from [12].

	Intra (CVw) and inter (CVg) individual biological variation *		Individuality index ((II) and Reference Change Value (RCV $_{95\%}$)**	
	CVw%	CVg%	II%	RCV $_{95\%}$
s Calcium	1.9	2.8	0.67	5.9
u Calcium	27.6	36.6	0.75	85.2
Ionized Calcium	1.7	2.2	0.77	5.3
s Phosphate	8.5	9.4	0.9	26.3
u Phosphate	26.4	26.5	1.0	81.8
s Creatinine	5.3	14.2	0.4	13.3
u Creatinine	24.0	24.5	1.0	74.4
Cr-clearance	13.6	13.0	1.0	42.1
s BAP	6.2	35.6	0.17	19.9
s C-Telopeptide	9.6	30.6	0.3	25.7
s Pancreatic Amylase	11.7	29.9	0.4	36.3

The usefulness of population reference intervals for diagnosing individual patient are limited when the individuality index (II) is less than 0.6 and acceptable when the II is greater than 1.4.

The difference between 2 serial results is significant and could be biologically relevant (change in health status) when it is greater than Reference Change Value (RCV $_{95\%}$), calculated as critical difference from biological variation of the analyte [12].

Ionized calcium is measured with ISE in whole blood (i.e. heparinized blood). For measuring iCa, caution is necessary to avoid loss of CO_2 that will increase pH and free Ca^{++} from proteins. Because pH affects calcium binding to albumin and subsequently the concentration of iCa, it has been suggested to correct "free" calcium concentration for pH: for each decline of 0.1 pH unit, iCa approximately increases by 0.05 mmol/L [11]. Moreover, heparin itself causes a 0.01 mmol/L decrease in iCa for each unit added per mL of blood (Table **7**).

Syringes containing dry heparin, "balanced" with electrolytes to minimize the binding of calcium to heparin, allowing anaerobic collection of blood, and minimizing effects of incomplete filling, are available. Blood should quickly be analyzed or centrifuged within 1-2 hours to prevent metabolic activity of cells during storage, which may affect both pH and iCa [1]. Ionized calcium concentrations are high at birth, decline by 10-20% after 1-3 days, then stabilize at concentrations slightly higher than in adults after 1 week (Table **1**). Differences in specimen preparation and electrode selectivity are probably responsible for differences in reported reference ranges (1.15-1.32 mmol/L). Desirable CVa and B are 0.9% and 0.7%, respectively, and reference change value (RCV $_{95\%}$) is 5.3 (Tables 5.8 and

5.9). Although the quality specifications are more stringent than tCa, ISE methods for iCa are able to reach the desirable goals of analytic performance [11].

Abundant evidence [6] establishes the importance of iCa in several pathologic conditions, such as critical care setting (i.e. severe hypercalcemia), outpatients with chronic kidney disease, suspected hyperparathyroidism, and MEN 1, although its direct measurement remains costly and technically challenging. For urinary calcium (uCa) measurement [10], the 24-h urine should be collected in a bottle containing 10 mL of HCl (6 mol/L), or acidified after collection to pH<2.0 for dissolving calcium salts (Table **6**).

The values in both healthy and sick individuals range widely, since calcium and protein intake modulate calcium excretion, as well as the phosphate excretion. In case of an average calcium diet (800 mg/day), uCa reference range is 2.50-7.50 mmol/day (100-300 mg/day). However, it lowers to 1.25-3.75 mmol/day in a low calcium diet, and falls to 0.13-1.00 mmol/day in a calcium-free diet (Tables 5.8 and 5.9).

Urinary calcium may be measured in random urine, and its concentration expressed as mmol/L, or preferably as mmol/g creatinine (mg/g Cr), with a reference range of 0.30-6.10 mmol/g Cr in males, and 0.225-8.20 mmol/ g Cr in females. The rate of calcium excretion can also be expressed as a calcium/creatinine (Ca/Cr) ratio. In healthy individuals, urinary Ca/Cr is usually <0.40 (when both analytes are expressed in mmol/L), and values >0.57 suggest hypercalciuria. Since about one third of patients with primary HPT have normal uCa output, the test has little value in differential diagnosis [11], and 2008 WAPHP [9] no longer suggests hypercalciuria (>10 mmol/day) as an indication for parathyroid surgery. However, uCa measurement is important for diagnosing FBHH, but in this case a more accurate test, such as the Ca/Cr ratio (normal value >0.02), is recommended [8].

Phosphate (inorganic phosphorus) is measured colorimetrically [10], in the fasting state, avoiding hemolysis and venous stasis, and separating from erythrocytes within 1 h after collection (Table **7**). The reference range is 0.71-1.45 mmol/L, while desirable CVa and B are 4.3% and 3.2%, respectively [5]. The analytic performance is usually accurate (Tables 5.8 and 5.9). Hypophosphatemia, defined as phosphate levels below 0.81 mmol/L, is found in about half of cases of primary HPT, but this neither confirms nor excludes the diagnosis. Hypophosphatemia may complicate MAH at any stage of the disease, and should be monitored routinely.

Serum (sCr) and urinary (uCr) creatinine, creatinine clearance (Cr-clearance), and glomerular filtration rate (GFR) are traditionally measured [10] by Jaffè reaction (alkaline picrate solution). This is affected by several interferences from many non-creatinine chromogens, and also is sensitive to pH and temperature changes. Technical modifications (kinetic method) improved the quality of this test, but more reliable enzymatic methods (based on measurement of ammonia generated when creatinine is hydrolyzed by creatinine-iminohydrolase) are available. The reference range varies according to gender, age, body muscle mass, and technique used (Table **10**).

Table 10: Reference range of serum creatinine according to different laboratory techniques and gender in adults (mg/dL).

Gender	Jaffè method	Kinetic method	Enzymatic method
Male	0.8-1.5	0.8-1.3	0.62-1.10
Female	0.7-1.4	0.6-1.2	0.45-0.75

On the basis of biological variation, desirable analytical specifications are the followings: CVa 2.7% and 12.0%, B 3.8% and 8.6%, and RCV$_{95\%}$ 13.3 and 74.4, for sCr and uCr, respectively [5]. The analytic performance is adequate (Tables 5.8 and 5.9).

Serum creatinine is usually measured to estimate renal function, but its relation to glomerular filtration rate (GFR) is a parabolic curve, and its plasma value remains within the normal range until more than

50% of renal function is lost. According to sCr levels, the stages of renal failure have been defined as follows: moderate (2.5-4.9 mg/dL), severe (5.0-9.9 mg/dL), and end-stage (10 mg/dL or greater).

For many years, the standard clinical tool for estimating GFR has been the measurement of Cr-clearance, based on the simultaneous determinations of sCr, uCr on a 24-h sample, and urinary volume (V), by the following formula:

$$Cr\text{-}clearance = uCr \times V/sCr$$

The result should be standardized to 1.73 m^2 body surface area (BSA), using a BSA table obtained from a nomogram based on weight and height of subjects. Reference range varies with age: in male and female of 20-40 years they span from 59 to 140 mL/min, and from 71 to 121 mL/min, respectively. For each decade after, values decrease about 6.5 mL/min [10]. Desirable CVa, B and RCV$_{95\%}$ are 6.8%, and 4.8% and 42.1, respectively [5]. To estimate renal impairment, values of standardized Cr-clearance (mL/min/1.73 m^2) were proposed as follows: borderline (62-80), slight (52-63), mild (42-52), moderate (28-42), and marked (<28). Advantages and disadvantages of 24-h rather than timed (2-h) urine collections were discussed with regard to the accuracy of collection and the reliability of the sample (Table **7**).

Several shortcuts to estimate GFR without collecting urine have been proposed. Since 2003, the National Kidney Foundation Kidney Disease Outcomes Quality Initiative (KDOQI) no longer recommends [14] the use of 24-h urinary collections for Cr-clearance, but the estimation of GFR from equations based on anthropometric criteria (i.e. factors affecting creatinine metabolism, such as age, gender, race, and weight) and serum measurements (creatinine, albumin, urea nitrogen), namely Cockcroft-Gault formula, and Modification of Diet in Renal Disease study (MDRD) equation n.7. The Cockcroft-Gault formula takes into account age (years), gender, body weight (kg) and sCr (mg/dL), but tends to overestimate GFR when compared to reference renal clearance (^{125}I-iothalamate):

$$Cr\text{-}clearance \ (mL/min) = (140\text{-}age) \times weight \times (0.85 \ if \ female) \ / \ (72 \times sCr)$$

MDRD equation n.7 takes into account age (years), gender, race, sCr (mg/dL), albumin (mg/dL), and urea nitrogen (sUN, mg/dL), but does not seem to overestimate GFR, when compared to the reference method. The eGFR (mL/min × 1.73 m^2) is obtained by the following formula:

$$170 \times (sCr)^{-0.999} \times (sUN)^{-0.170} \times (Alb)^{+0.318} \times (Age)^{-0.176} \times (0.762 \ if \ female) \times (1.180 \ if \ African \ American)$$

The 2008 WAPHPT guidelines [9] recommend the use of the MDRD equation n.7 as the most accurate tool for estimating GFR. Another easier MDRD equation is often used: it takes into account only sCr and some anthropomorphic data (age, gender, race). The eGFR (mL/min × 1.73 m^2) is obtained by the following formula:

$$186 \ or \ 175 \times (sCr)^{-1.154} \times (Age)^{-0.203} \times (0.742 \ if \ female) \times (1.210 \ if \ African \ American)$$

The factor 186 should be used by traditional Jaffè method users, while factor 175 by the laboratories using the enzymatic method or methods calibrated to the NIST (The National Institute of Standards and Technology) standard. Some limitations exist in the diagnostic use of the latter equation, such as in younger subjects (<18 years) and in patients with eGFR >60 mL/min/1.73 m^2. The National Kidney Disease Education Program (NKDEP) recommends [14] that values >60 mL/min/1.73 m^2 be reported as "greater than 60". Since the decision limits for chronic kidney disease (CKD) was defined as < 60 mL/min/1.73 m^2, and for kidney failure as <15 mL/min/1.73 m^2, the second MDRD equation allows a safe diagnosis and an accurate following of the course of CKD. Thus, NKDEP [14] recommends its use in adults with CKD, and in those at risk for CKD (diabetes, hypertension, and family history of kidney failure). Routine reporting of eGFR by laboratories is recommended, but often it is not carried out. Clinicians should be aware of the methods and formulas used by their local laboratory.

SPECIFIC LABORATORY FINDINGS

PTH, the linear amino-acid peptide produced in the parathyroid glands, is present simultaneously in peripheral blood as intact PTH(1-84), and as a heterogeneous group of peptide fragments, not only in healthy subjects but also in patients affected by primary and secondary HPT. Indeed, the concentration of peptide fragments is several-fold greater than that of the intact hormone. Some of these fragments arise from the metabolism of PTH(1-84) in various tissues, most notably liver, while others are released from the parathyroid glands directly, reflecting the intracellular degradation of the hormone. The identification and quantification of PTH-derived peptides in plasma is the major obstacle to the development of reliable PTH assays, because some of these peptides interacted with the immunoassays used to determine PTH levels [15].

Most of what we know on PTH bioactivity has been associated with the amino-sequence 1-34 of the PTH structure, which acts on the type 1 PTH receptor (PTH-1) [16]. This knowledge has influenced the evolution of the PTH assays. In the last 45 years, several PTH assays have been made available, after the first radioimmunoassay (RIA) for human PTH, proposed by Berson *et al.* in 1963, that initiated a new era in the diagnosis of parathyroid diseases. These competitive immunoassays (IMAs), now defined as "first-generation" IMAs, used multivalent antibodies raised against parathyroid extracts of various species (mainly bovine and human), PTH(1-84) preparations with various degrees of purity or synthetic peptides as standards, and purified ^{125}I-PTH(1-84) or ^{125}I-PTH fragments as tracers. The main epitopes recognized by these assays were in the C-terminal (amino acids 53-84) and in mid C-terminal (amino acids 44-68) domains. Only 20% of the immunoreactivity detected by these first generation assays was similar or identical to PTH(1-84), while the remaining 80% was due to smaller C-PTH fragments. These early assays differ widely from one another: they show different reference ranges, and are unable to distinguish non-parathyroid from parathyroid hypercalcemia, due to the presence of C-PTH fragments, which are present in both clinical conditions [16].

For these reasons, these assays were substituted in the '80s by the non-competitive "two-site" immunoassays (called "second-generation" IMAs), which are based on two distinct antibodies that recognize two different epitopes: one N-terminal (1-34), and other C-terminal (39-84). However, these methods measure only the intact PTH. The introduction of dual-antibody immunoassays circumvented many of the shortcomings of single-antibody RIAs. The original two-site immunoradiometric (IRMA) assay (Nichols Institute), with a reference range of 12 to 65 mg/L, constituted the standard method for the definition of various guidelines proposed in the literature. Now it is no longer available and it has been replaced by numerous second-generation assays, which produce PTH values that vary widely between 50% and 150% of the expected Nichols PTH values. This variability made problematic the diagnosis of PHPT, using 65 ng/L as a cut-off value [17].

The meaning of intact PTH included the notion of bioactive PTH, i.e. PTH capable of binding and activating a PTH-1 receptor. Therefore, some investigations provided data suggesting that other molecular forms, specifically N-terminal truncated PTH-derived fragments [4,7,10,15-84(PTH)], called non-(1-84)PTH fragments, were also measured by the available second-generation IRMAs. These fragments accounted for up to 20 % in normal individuals and for up to 50% of PTH immunoreactivity in renal failure patients. The fragment PTH(7-84) was demonstrated to cause hypocalcemia, and to antagonize PTH(1-34) and PTH(1-84), having inhibitory effects on bone resorption: this suggests a dual control of calcium concentration via N- and C-PTH molecular forms.

To overcome these limitations, the "third-generation" IMAs were proposed, with the amino-terminal specific antibody directed against the first four amino-terminal amino acids, fundamental for the activation of the PTH-1 receptor (Fig. **3**).

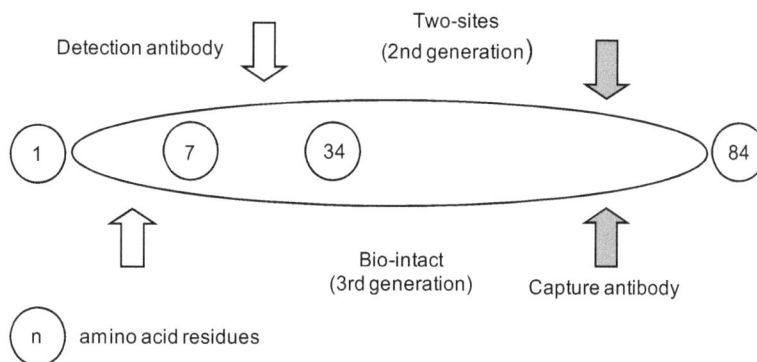

Figure 3: Second- and third-generations of PTH assays. Modified from [17]

The introduction of these methods for the detection of PTH(1-4) opened a new chapter in this field of study. The reference range of these methods is from 7 to 36 ng/L. These last immunoassays also permit an indirect evaluation of non-(1-84) PTH fragments by subtracting a third-generation PTH value from a second-generation PTH value and the calculation of a PTH(1-84)/non-(1-84) PTH ratio [17].

According to the 2008 WAPHPT [9], some recommendations for PTH measurement should be made. In spite of the considerable interest for the comprehension of PTH physiology, the third-generation PTH assays are not yet proven to be superior to the second-generation assays in clinical practice. Currently, there is no recommendation to switch from second- to third-generation assays. Because the two generation PTH assays are usually highly correlated, significant differences in the clinical information provided by these methods are unlikely, and their clinical sensitivity in detecting elevated PTH values is similar.

Reference ranges should be established for serum PTH in vitamin D replete healthy individuals, because vitamin deficiency or insufficiency causes PTH elevation, as demonstrated in different groups of patients, such as elderly, African American individuals, low calcium intake patients and obese subjects. This approach causes a 30% reduction in the upper limit of PTH reference values of second- and third-generation IMAs (from 65 to 45 ng/L, and from 45 to 35 ng/L, respectively) [18]. The analytical quality goals for PTH, based on biological variation, should be 6% for imprecision and 12% for accuracy, usually reached by laboratory methods. Strict attention to the technique of blood drawing, in particular the use of a catheter, is mandatory to prevent contamination and avoid spurious PTH test results [19]. A specified collection method for PTH immunoassay using EDTA or citrate plasma is recommended [20].

The measurement of circulating 25(OH)D in either serum or plasma is considered the best clinical indicator of vitamin D status, widely used for the diagnosis vitamin D deficiency or insufficiency, and the prescription of vitamin D supplementation [18]. The important forms of vitamin D are vitamin D_3 (cholecalciferol) and vitamin D_2 (ergocalciferol). These 2 forms of vitamin D are carried in the blood as a complex with a vitamin D-binding protein: once in the circulation, vitamin D is hydroxylated to 25(OH)D in the liver. More than 95% of 25(OH)D measurable in serum is typically 25(OH)D_3, while 25(OH)D_2 reaches measurable concentrations only in patients taking vitamin D supplementation [21] (see Chapter 1).

The serum levels of 25(OH)D are often reduced in patients with primary HPT and may mask hypercalcemia in some patients, mimicking normocalcemic HPT. Various manual IMAs that employ vitamin D antibodies for analytic measurement are available for quantifying circulating 25(OH)D_2 and 25(OH)D_3. Several methods have been described that use high-pressure liquid chromatography (HPLC) with ultraviolet detection and liquid chromatography-tandem mass spectrometry (LC-MS/MS). The use of these three technologies revealed substantial and significant variability between laboratories in a recent vitamin D external quality assessment programme [22].

Due to the recently discovered important role of vitamin D deficiency as a risk factor not only for bone metabolism diseases, but also for many common and serious diseases, including cancer, diabetes mellitus and cardiovascular diseases, there is an emerging need for automation of vitamin D assays, with improved output and efficiency. Recently, two commercial direct automated immunoassays specific for 25(OH)D$_3$ measurement based on electro chemiluminescence (CLIA) detection have been introduced [21]. The following recommendations for 25(OH)D measurement may be offered [18].

Due to a significant prevalence of vitamin D insufficiency in patients with primary HPT and the benefits of vitamin D supplementation, it is recommended that 25(OH)D concentrations be measured in all patients with HPT-related hypercalcemia. Precise measurement of serum levels of 25(OH)D remains a challenge, because the above-described inter-method and inter-laboratory variability makes clinical assessment of vitamin D status of patients problematic. The intra- and interassay variability is much greater at low levels compared with high levels of serum 25(OH)D. A modest systematic bias between methods (RIA, CLIA, HPLC, LC-MS/MS) was recently observed at a 25(OH)D concentration of 30 ng/mL, but the use of a set of calibrators, standardized against a reference material, will enhance inter-laboratory agreement [22]. The National Institute of Standards and Technology (NIST) recently developed a standard reference material (SRM 972) for these purposes [23]. An international consensus on a reference range for 25(OH)D levels in healthy subjects and in patients with primary HPT has not yet been achieved. For several authors, the optimal level is considered to be the concentration below which PTH levels begin to rise [24]. Estimates of this optimal level vary widely (from 30 to 110 nmol/L, or 8-44 ng/mL), but the largest and most convincing study would suggest a level of 75-80 nmol/L, or 30 ng/mL [21]. As a consequence, there is an increasing clinical consensus that values less than this cut-off point are indicative of suboptimal vitamin D status. The desirable 25(OH)D levels in the population are between 90-120 nmol/L or 36-48 ng/mL, and an intake of 1000-2000 IU (12-25 µg) of vitamin D for all adults is needed. No special specimen type or blood drawing procedure are recommended for 25(OH)D testing [24].

PTHrP was identified in 1987 as a tumor product (polypeptide of 139-173 amino acids and molecular weight approximately 17 kDa), that mimics certain action of PTH. PTHrP and PTH are products of two different genes, but they have similar primary and secondary structures (particularly in the first 13 amino acids of the N-terminal domain) in regions important for PTH receptor binding and activation. Thus, the two polypeptides share a comparable secondary structure that binds similarly to PTH-1 receptor, also called PTH/PTHrP receptor [25].

A large number of immunoassays for PTHrP have been developed using antibodies directed against N-terminal, midmolecule and C-terminal sequences, as well as "two-site" assays spanning N-terminal and midmolecule sequences (RIAs, IRMAs, CLIAs). Clear recommendations for PTHrP measurement are not yet available, and there are no published guidelines regarding the utilization of PTHrP in hypercalcemic patients. Due to the low diagnostic sensitivity (30-35%) and high specificity (>95%), the use of PTHrP testing in the assessment of hypercalcemia is of limited value, and is more appropriately performed after the measurement of PTH. In case of low o low-normal (<30 ng/L) PTH level, the measurement of PTHrP should be obtained only when the cause of hypercalcemia is not readily apparent. The reference values range from 0 (undetectable) to 2.0 pmol/L, depending on the analytical sensitivity of the immunoassay methods which range from 2.0 pmol/L (early RIAs) to 0.1 pmol/L (recent IRMAs and CLIA). The recommended collection method for PTHrP immunoassay is EDTA plasma with protease inhibitors [25].

Since PTH activates both osteoclasts and osteoblasts, bone turnover formation markers, such as total alkaline phosphatase (ALP), bone-specific alkaline phosphatase (BAP) and osteocalcin, as well as bone turnover resorption markers, including urinary pyridinium cross-links pyridinoline (PYD), deoxypyridoline (DPD), collagen cross-link-associated C-telopeptide (CTx), and collagen cross-link-associated N-telopeptide (NTx), are increased (Tables 5.8 and 5.9).

ALP is not an accurate tool for assessment of bone turnover, because changes in serum concentration within the normal range of values may be significant for an increase of bone formation. The immunometric determination of BAP is the method of choice for evaluating osteoblasts activity. BAP has several advantages over osteocalcin for biological and technical reasons: BAP does not exhibit diurnal variation because of its long half-life (1-3 days) and is more stable in vitro and does not require special specimen handling [25]. However, BAP may be misleading in individuals with liver disease, where a hepatic isoform of BAP cross-reacts in the assay, or with severe osteomalacia, where BAP increases but fails to mineralize.

The pyridinium cross-links are released with type I collagen degradation, and can be assayed in urine using either a random specimen or a timed collection. Their diurnal variations in excretion should be considered, and marker levels are highest in the early morning, and lowest in the afternoon. A second morning void is usually recommended. Using serum to measure telopeptides increases convenience, eliminates the need to measure urine creatinine, and reduces within-subject and day-to-day variation [10].

Since the 1990s, several reports emphasized the role of biochemical markers of bone turnover in cancer patients, for predicting metastatic bone disease and monitoring the efficacy of antiresorptive therapy, but these reports are not fully convincing. Indeed, the usefulness of bone markers as predictive of the likelihood of bone loss or fractures in patients with untreated primary HPT is still unclear.

The value of gene testing analysis in the assessment of genetic syndromes leading to hypercalcemia has been addressed after gene sequencing techniques are available from many laboratories. According to the 2008 WAPHPT guidelines [9], genetic testing has several different roles: (1) confirming a syndrome in a proband, (2) determining the zone of sequence that can be shared with relatives, (3) individuating carriers among asymptomatic relatives, (4) monitoring known carriers for emergence of potentially morbid syndromal tumors, and (5) defining indications for more aggressive therapy (i.e. prophylactic surgery in MEN 2 syndrome). In the presence of mild (<3.0 mmol/L) hypercalcemia, FBHH syndrome should be suspected if serum PTH level is around normal and the patient is hypocalciuric (Ca-Cr clearance ratio <0.01). FBHH is a rare autosomal dominant disease caused by a deactivating mutation of CASR in both parathyroid glands and kidney cells, resulting in an increase of the set-point value for inhibition of PTH secretion. Patients with FBHH have normal PTH suppressibility during *in vivo* calcium infusion [8].

The homozygous form results in severe neonatal hyperparathyroidism. Heterozygotes are usually asymptomatic, with incidental mild hypercalcemia, decreased urinary calcium excretion, an inappropriately normal or mildly elevated PTH, and a mild to moderate increase in serum magnesium. It is important to distinguish this disorder from primary HPT, because these patients do not benefit by parathyroidectomy or calcium-lowering therapy. Age at diagnosis, absence of symptoms and classical complications of primary HPT, and PTH assay are useful indicators, but it may be a challenge to make this distinction when both serum and urinary calcium and PTH levels overlap those of HPT patients (Table **2**).

Genetic testing with sequencing of calcium receptor gene is commercially available, and is necessary to make the diagnosis in heterozygotes. However, about 30% of families do not have an identifiable CASR mutation.

At present, four hereditary syndromes are known that may result in development of primary HPT: (1) multiple endocrine neoplasia type 1 (MEN 1) and (2) type 2A (MEN 2A), (3) hyperparathyroidism-jaw tumor (HPT-JT) syndrome, and (4) familial isolated primary HPT (FIPH), which seems to be an early stage of MEN 1 or HPT-JT. Except the latter, these syndromes are characterized by combined occurrence of tumors in many different tissues, with some specific clusters. These clinical constellations, when present, and the young age of patients, are suggestive as a diagnosis of familial primary HPT. In MEN 1 syndrome, MEN 1 gene analysis fails in about 30% of cases, due in part to a mutation of p27 gene [8].

The main role of genetic testing in MEN 1 is to give long-term information to patients, relatives, and care providers. In MEN 2, the RET oncogene testing is of value in considering prophylactic thyroidectomy to prevent the development of medullary thyroid carcinoma. HPT-JT syndrome is very rare, but HRPT2 testing in relatives can result in the identification and surveillance of individuals at risk for parathyroid cancer. FIPH syndrome has no specific features, and some cases represent occult presentation of one of the above mentioned syndromes. Testing of CASR, MEN1 and HRPT2 does not detect any mutations in less than 20% of suspected cases. The expense is substantial, but the implications for the proband and the family can be reasons to recommend genetic testing in these patients.

In conclusion, according to the 2008 WAPHPT guidelines [9], DNA sequence testing for mutations of CASR, MEN1 and HRPT2 genes can provide useful information in familial hypercalcemia, but is not recommended on a routine basis. Mutations in the RET gene are important in the management of medullary thyroid carcinoma in MEN 2A. It is important to note that only a positive test has to be considered for clinical diagnosis, because of the high rate of false negative results.

MONITORING COMPLICATIONS OF HYPERCALCEMIA & DRUG THERAPY

In many cases the distinction between symptoms and complications of hypercalcemia is unclear or arbitrary. Signs and symptoms relate both to the severity of hypercalcemia and to the rapid rate of its rise. Severe hypercalcemia is always symptomatic ("bones, stones, abdominal groans, and psychic moans") and requires hospitalization, because patients can present life threatening complications, such as acute pancreatitis, acute renal failure, and coma.

In evaluating renal function, sCr and/or eGFR are useful tools for diagnosing and following the renal failure. Relationship between hypercalcemia and pancreatitis is controversial. Nevertheless, in the diagnosis of acute pancreatitis it is useful to determine serum amylase, or, preferably, the specific pancreatic isoform that avoids enzymatic activity from salivary isoform (Tables 5.8 and 5.9).

In patients with acute hypercalcemia, repeated serum calcium measurements are the main tool for monitoring treatment, which consists of restoring renal function, rehydration with saline in combination with loop diuretics, and bisphosphonates administration (see Chapter 4). Serum calcium levels begin to fall within 12-24 hours after therapy is started, reaching the nadir (normal calcemia) at 48-72 hours. This should remain in the normal or near-normal range for 1-3 weeks (see Chapter 8). Because of potential nephrotoxicity of bisphosphonates, a careful monitoring of renal function is required. In nonresponders, in lack of specific guidelines, the suggested criteria leading to hemodialysis treatment includes a Cr-clearance falling below 10-20 mL/min, congestive heart failure, or both [2].

Depending on the cause of hypercalcemia, several alterations may occur, affecting mainly bones and kidney. The skeleton is best evaluated by bone mineral density (BMD), whereas bone biochemical markers may be helpful in monitoring this, although there are several limitations mentioned above [26]. Because the filtered load of calcium is increased, and despite the PTH-induced increase in renal tubule calcium ion resorption, patients with HPT frequently present hypercalciuria, often resulting in nephrolithiasis and nephrocalcinosis (see Chapter 1).

Once the diagnosis of primary HPT is made, the surgical treatment should be considered. The 2008 WAPHPT [9] defined guidelines for parathyroidectomy, that include ages <50 years old, iCa, PTH, eGFR, as well as BMD measurement, but excluded a 24-hour urine calcium collection, modifying the old 2002 guidelines [7]. Chapter 7 discusses the questions related to the surgical treatment of HPT.

In surgical management of HPT, intraoperative measurements of PTH can help surgeons remove a more precise amount of parathyroid tissue. In cases of single adenoma, successful parathyroidectomy is confirmed when the PTH falls by 50% or more from baseline, approximately 10 minutes following complete resection of hyperfunctioning parathyroid tissue. This takes place because of the very short half-life of PTH (<5 min). Different limits (40%, 65%, 75%) have been reported, but they are derived from limited studies [27]. At surgery, a pre-incision baseline PTH specimen should be obtained. With the aim of reducing the number of false-negative results, a second pre-excision specimen is suggested in patients with identified single parathyroid adenoma, considering the highest PTH value as the baseline (Fig. **4**).

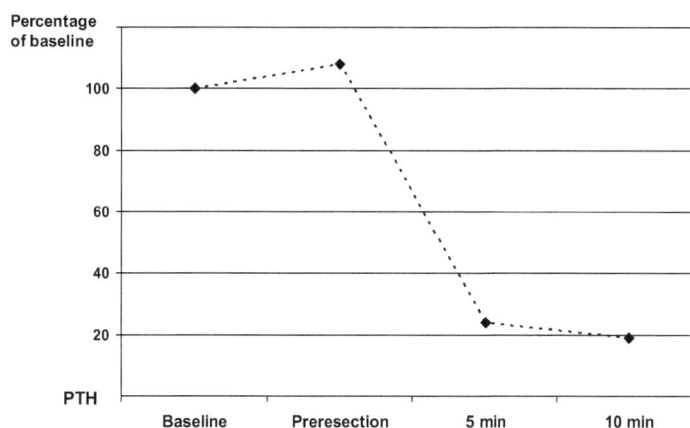

Figure 4: Intraoperative PTH concentrations during parathyroidectomy. Modified from [27].

If the PTH does not decline sufficiently after parathyroidectomy, a further cervical exploration is mandatory. The intraoperative PTH is particularly helpful in cases of reoperation and in ectopic location of parathyroid glands [27].

According to the 2008 WAPHPT guidelines [9], patients who do not meet the criteria for surgery, are treated conservatively and followed longitudinally (Table **11**) with regular (annual) assessment of tCa, Cr, and 3-sites BMD every 1-2 years, while 24-h uCa and Cr-clearance are no longer recommended, modifying the indications in the 2002 guidelines [7].

Table 11: Management guidelines for patients with asymptomatic primary hyperparathyroidism who did not undergo parathyroidectomy. Adapted from [9].

Parameters	Suggestions
Serum calcium	Annually
24-h urine calcium	Not recommended
Creatinine clearance (24-h urine collections)	Not recommended
Serum creatinine	Annually
Bone density	Every 1-2 yr (3 sites)
Abdominal X-ray (±ultrasound)	Not recommended

In patients with MAH, tCa, Cr and serum phosphate levels should be followed closely, with the goals of keeping serum phosphate in the range of 0.98-1 mmol/L, Cr in the normal range, and the calcium-phosphate product below 40 (ideally 30), when both are expressed in mmol/L [2]. It is important to note that hypophosphatemia may develop in most MAH patients at some point during the course of the disease. The presence of several pathologic and therapeutic factors increases the difficulty of treating hypercalcemia [13]. Monitoring tCa after medications are discontinued is also necessary to confirm diagnosis and recovery in hypercalcemia associated to lithium (2 to 4 weeks) and to thiazides (2-3 months) [11]. In patients with non-PTH mediated hypercalcemia of unknown etiology, baseline laboratory investigations should include full blood count (CBC), renal and liver function tests, ESR or C-reactive protein, and serum and urine protein electrophoresis. Some authors add also electrolytes and serum magnesium concentration, but these are not necessary unless specifically indicated [4]. Moreover, serum magnesium is a poor indicator of physiologic active intracellular magnesium concentration.

CONCLUSIONS

In mild, moderate, and severe hypercalcemia, laboratory findings are essential in discovering, assessing and monitoring the course and therapy of the disease. The main tools are some standard biochemical tests able to assess calcium balance (tCa, iCa, uCa, phosphate) and renal function (sCr, Cr-clearance, eGFR), and some specific biochemical tests, such as iPTH, 25(OH)D, and genetic sequencing, used to clarify the cause of hypercalcemia and, subsequently, to determine appropriate therapy. Of the standard tests, the best indicator for calcium imbalance is iCa, because it correctly defines "hypercalcemia". For renal function, sCr and derived eGFR are the tests of choice, according to the recent WAPHPT guidelines.

The measurement of iPTH, determined by a second- or third-generation method, is the key test in the diagnostic algorithm of hypercalcemia, together with 25(OH)D and tests of renal function for detecting secondary HPT or renal complications of hypercalcemia. Ca-Cr clearance ratio is useful for FBHH diagnosis. Calcium and renal function tests (eGFR, sCr) are recommended for referring patients for surgery as well as for monitoring asymptomatic HPT patients. Intraoperative iPTH is helpful if parathyroidectomy is performed, while genetic testing are indicated only as a second step study, in patients with familial HPT.

In MAH, iCa is the test of choice for monitoring effects of medical therapy, while 25(OH)D may be helpful in differential diagnosis with granulomatous diseases, and serum phosphate is used in monitoring the course of hypercalcemia. PTHrP testing is not routinely recommended, and should be required only after measuring PTH.

REFERENCES

[1]   Toffaletti JG. Blood Gases and Electrolytes. 2nd Ed. Washington, DC: AACC Press 2009.
[2]   Stewart AF. Hypercalcemia associated with cancer. N Engl J Med 2005; 352: 373-379.
[3]   Slomp J, van der Voort PHJ, Gerritsen RT, Berk JAM, Bakker AJ. Albumin-adjusted calcium is not suitable for diagnosis of hyper- and hypocalcemia in the critically ill. Crit Care Med 2003; 31: 1389-1393.
[4]   Smellie WSA, Vanderpump MPJ, Fraser WD, Bowley R, Shaw N. Best practice in primary care pathology: review 11. J Clin Pathol 2008; 61: 410-8.
[5]   http://www.westgard.com (accessed 10.08.2009)
[6]   Calvi LM, Bushinsky DA. When is it appropriate to order ionized calcium? J Am Soc Nephrol 2008; 19: 1257-1260.
[7]   Bilezikian JP, Potts JT Jr, Fuleihan GEH, *et al*. Summary statement from a Workshop on asymptomatic Primary Hyperparathyroidism: a perspective for the 21st century. J Clin Endocrinol Metab 2002; 87: 5353-5361.
[8]   Töke J, Patócs A, Balogh K, *et al*. Parathyroid hormone-dependent hypercalcemia. Wien Klin Wochenschhr 2009; 121: 236-245.
[9]   Bilezikian JP, Khan AA, Potts JT. Guidelines for the management of asymptomatic primary hyperparathyroidism: summary statement from the third international workshop. J Clin Endocrinol Metab 2009; 94: 335-339.
[10]   Wu AHB. Tietz Clinical Guide to Laboratory Tests. 4th Ed. St. Louis: WB Saunders Company 2006.
[11]   Younes NA, Shafagoj Y, Khatib F, Ababneh M. Laboratory screening for hyperparathyroidism. Clin Chim Acta 2005; 353: 1-12.
[12]   Ricós C, Cava F, Garcia-Lario JV, *et al*. The reference change value: a proposal to interpret laboratory reports in serial testing based on biological variation. Scand J Clin Lab Invest 2004; 64:175-184.
[13]   Lumachi F, Brunello A, Roma A, Basso U. Cancer-induced hypercalcemia. Anticancer Res 2009; 29: 1551-1556.
[14]   National Kidney Foundation. KDOQI clinical practice guidelines for bone metabolism and disease in chronic kidney disease. Am J Kidney Dis 2003; 42: S1-S200.

[15] Friedman PA, Goodman WG. PTH (1-84)/PTH (7-84): a balance of power. Am J Physiol Renal Physiol 2006; 290: F975-F984.

[16] D'Amour P. Circulating PTH molecular forms: what we know and what we don't. Kidney Int 2006; 102 (suppl.1): S29-S33.

[17] Cole DE, Webb S, Chan PC. Update on parathyroid hormone: new tests and new challenges for external quality assessment. Clin Biochem 2007; 40: 585-590.

[18] Eastell R, Arnold A, Brandi ML, *et al.* Diagnosis of asymptomatic primary hyperparathyroidism: proceedings of the third international workshop. J Clin Endocrinol Metab 2009; 94: 340-530.

[19] Viljoen A, Singh DK, Twomey PJ, Farrington K. Analytical quality goals for parathyroid hormone based on biological variation. Clin Chem Lab Med 2008; 46: 1438-1442.

[20] Joly D, Drueke TB, Alberti C, *et al.* Variation in serum and plasma PTH levels in second-generation assays in hemodialysis patients: a cross-sectional study. Am J Kidney Dis 2008; 51: 987-995.

[21] Dawson-Hughes B, Heaney RP, Holick MF, Lips P, Meunier PJ, Vieth R. Estimates of optimal vitamin D status. Osteoporosis Int 2005; 16: 713-716.

[22] Binkley N, Kruger D, Gemar D, Drezner MK. Correlation among 25-hydroxyvitamin D assays. J Clin Endocrinol Metab 2008; 93:1804-1808.

[23] Phinney KW. Development of a standard reference material for vitamin D in serum. Am J Clin Nutr 2008; 88 (suppl.): 511S-512S.

[24] Bischoff-Ferrari HA. Optimal serum 25-hydroxyvitamin D levels for multiple health outcomes. Adv Exp Med Biol 2008; 624: 55-71.

[25] Fritchie K, Zedek D, Grenache DG. The clinical utility of parathyroid hormone-related peptide in the assessment of hypercalcemia. Clin Chim Acta 2009; 402: 146-149.

[26] Lumachi F, Ermani M, Camozzi V, Tombolan V, Luisetto G. Changes of bone formation markers osteocalcin and bone-specific alkaline phosphatase in postmenopausal women with osteoporosis. Ann N Y Acad Sci 2009; 1173: E60-E63.

[27] Sokoll LJ, Wians FH Jr, Remaley AT. Rapid intraoperative immunoassay of parathyroid hormone and other hormones: a new paradigm for Point-of-Care Testing. Clin Chem 2004; 50: 1126-1135.

CHAPTER 6

Imaging Studies in Patients with Hypercalcemia

Grazia Guzzetta, Maria Guzzetta and Gianpietro Feltrin

Department of Radiology, University of Padua, School of Medicine, 35128 Padova, Italy

Abstract: In patients with hypercalcemia the usefulness and indications of imaging studies depend on the pathological condition causing the disease. The main causes of hypercalcemia are primary hyperparathyroidism (HPT) and malignancy, but an increased serum calcium level can also be the consequence of several diseases affecting different organs, being the object of specific imaging studies. Unfortunately, they are not able to confirm or exclude all those disorders, having the purpose to examine the morphology of each organ involved in the pathogenesis of hypercalcemia, such as parathyroid glands, kidneys and urinary tract, bones and other organs. In patients with HPT the aim of imaging studies is to localize the enlarged PT glands, both in patients with single PT adenoma, and in those with multiple glands disease. The first studies should be neck ultrasonography and sestamibi scintigraphy. If they are negative or discordant, ectopic PT glands are suspected, and computed tomography (CT) scan, magnetic resonance imaging (MR) and more recently positron emission tomography (PET) should be suggested. Ultrasonography has a good accuracy in the detection of renal stones, but unenhanced CT has the best sensitivity. In patients with bone metastases the first imaging technique to be used is whole body bone scintigraphy, followed by plan x-ray of single sites, while CT and MRI may complete the differential diagnosis. CT is usually suggested for mineralized and rib lesions, MRI is preferable for bone marrow lesions, while ^{18}F-fluoro-2-deoxyglucose (FDG)-PET is useful in the detection of soft tissue or bone metastases.

INTRODUCTION

Hypercalcemia is the result of the interaction of three mechanisms regulating calcium metabolism: (1) increased intestinal absorption, (2) increased bone resorption, and (3) decreased renal excretion. In patients with hypercalcemia the usefulness and indications of imaging studies depend on the pathological condition causing the disease. Thus, they should be selected according to the results of clinical and biochemical study of the patient and the differential diagnosis, that usually distinguishes between patients with primary hyperparathyroidism (HPT) and those with everything else [1].

The main causes of hypercalcemia are primary HPT and malignancy, but an increased serum calcium level can also be the consequence of several diseases affecting different organs, every disease being the object of specific imaging studies. Unfortunately, they are not able to confirm or exclude all those disorders, having the purpose to examine the morphology of each organ involved in the pathogenesis of hypercalcemia, such as parathyroid (PT) glands, kidneys and urinary tract, bones and other organs.

PARATHYROID GLANDS

Patients with symptomatic primary HPT, as well as those with asymptomatic HPT who meet surgical indications according to the 2009 Workshop Guidelines for the management of asymptomatic primary HPT [2], should undergo preoperative localization studies with the aim of shortening operative time, and reducing the rate of unsuccessful surgical explorations [3-4]. Primary HPT is usually caused by a solitary PT adenoma. Multiple-gland disease, such as hyperplasia or multiple adenomas, accounts for about 15% of cases, while hyperfunctioning PT carcinoma is an uncommon finding. Hyperparathyroidism also occurs as part of familial syndromes, including multiple endocrine neoplasia type 1 (MEN 1), type 2A (MEN 2A), familial isolated primary HPT, and HPT-jaw tumor syndromes. All of them typically causing hyperplasia of all PT glands (see Chapter 2).

Secondary HPT is the consequence of acute renal failure, virtually appearing when creatinine clearance is less than 20-40 mL/min, but may also occur both in patients with recovery from rhabdomyolysis and in those who underwent renal transplantation. Phosphate retention, together with increased calcitriol

Franco Lumachi & Stefano M.M. Basso (Eds)

[1,25(OH)$_2$D$_3$] production, represent the *stimuli* to all-gland hyperplasia. Tertiary HPT occurs rarely, as a consequence of severe secondary HPT, leading to unresponsive hyperfunction of the PT glands (see Chapter 1). Fig. **1** shows the preoperative imaging techniques available for localizing enlarged PT glands. High invasive studies are performed only in selected cases. Intraoperative methods are radioguided surgery, and intraoperative ultrasonography (see Chapter 7).

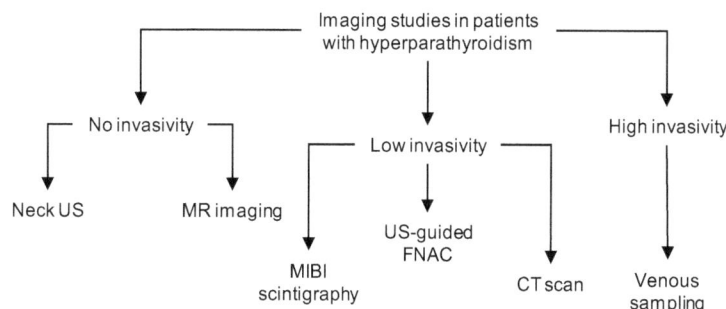

Figure 1: Preoperative imaging studies available for patients with hyperparathyroidism, according to their invasivity. US=ultrasonography, MR=magnetic resonance, MIBI=methoxyisobutilisonitrile, FNAC=fine-needle aspiration cytology, CT=computed tomography.

The aim of imaging studies is to localize the enlarged PT glands, both in patients with single PT adenoma, and in those with multiple glands disease. They are usually chosen according to the radiologist's experience, availability, and costs, but are also related to the type of surgical approach (i.e. unilateral *versus* bilateral, minimally-invasive *versus* traditional parathyroidectomy).

The anatomic distribution of the PT glands varies widely. There are four glands in approximately 85% of cases, more than four in 13%, and only three parathyroids in 2-3% of cases [5]. Moreover, the position of the glands is symmetrical in only 70-80% of cases.

Because of failure of descent, the superior glands can be situated higher up in the neck, while the inferior are frequently close to the lower thyroid pole, or in the upper thymus [5, 6]. The sites of more frequent ectopic locations of PT glands are reported in Table **1**. Parathyroid adenomas are not very large, and they can take rise in each of the PT glands (Fig. **2**).

Table 1: Main ectopic sites of the parathyroid glands.

Cervical	Extra-cervical (mediastinal)
Retrotracheal	*Retrotracheal*
Paraesophageal	*Paraesophageal*
Thyrothymic ligament	*Near the brachiocephalic veins & artery*
Intrathymic	*Pulmonary hilus & pericardium*

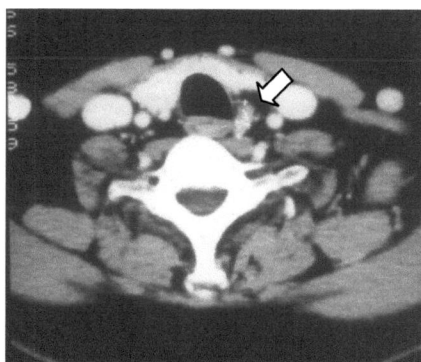

Figure 2: Contrast-enhanced helical computed tomography (CT) scanning image acquired 30 sec after nonionic contrast medium intravenous injection, showing a significantly enhanced paratracheal mass, in a 56-year-old

woman with primary hyperparathyroidism, corresponding to a parathyroid adenoma (arrow) of the left inferior parathyroid gland sited at the dorsal profile of the thyroid lobe.

Imaging studies are not useful in confirming diagnosis of primary HPT, exclusively based on serum laboratory tests results (see Chapter 5). Thus, in patients with persistent or recurrent HPT it is mandatory to reconfirm the diagnosis before surgical reexploration, as well as perform a careful localization study.

The information obtained by imaging studies are the following [7, 8]:

1. Preoperative identification and localization of hyperfunctioning PT glands before unilateral surgical exploration or minimally-invasive parathyroidectomy, both video-assisted and radioguided (see Chapter 7). Imaging studies are the sole way to differentiate between solitary PT adenoma and multiglandular disease causing HPT;

2. Localization of ectopic PT glands, especially in patients with persistent or recurrent HPT;

3. Identification of associated diseases, such as thyroid nodules or lymph nodes;

4. Definition of neck and mediastinum surgical anatomy.

Parathyroid glands originate from the third and fourth pharyngeal pouches, and are usually placed at the postero-internal surface of the thyroid lobe (Fig. **3**) (see Chapter 7). Due to their small (5-6 mm) size, they can be identified only by computed tomography (CT) scanning, while both magnetic resonance (MR) imaging and neck ultrasonography (US) are not able to visualize all normal glands.

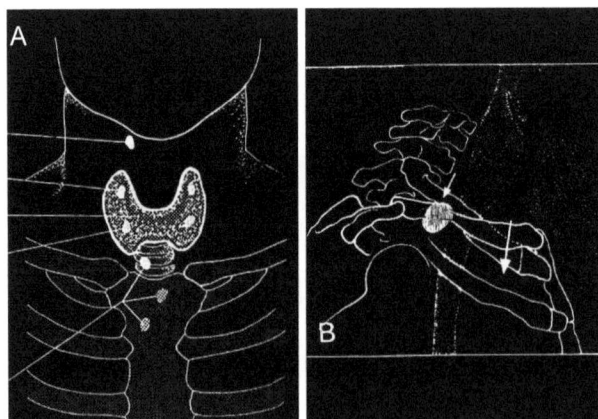

Figure 3: Typical location of the parathyroid glands, usually masked by the thyroid at scintigraphic scanning, and their more frequent ectopic locations. Scheme of possible location of ectopic parathyroid and thyroid tumors in anterior (A) and lateral (B) projections. Thyroid adenomas, originating from the third pharyngeal pouch, are usually anterior to the trachea, while parathyroid adenomas, originating from the fourth pharyngeal pouch, are located dorsally to the trachea.

Computed Tomography Scan

CT scan of the neck and mediastinum is usually performed after a non-ionic contrast intravenous administration, using speed (1 slice/0.8 sec, slice collimation 3-5 mm, pitch value 1.5) axial thin sections, and a frontal scout view identifying the upper limit of the heart, which was the lower region of interest and the first scan at CT examination [9].

Their rich vascularity allows the identification of abnormal PT tissues at CT scan even if the surrounding structures, such as thyroid gland, show high enhancement values, mimicking PT lesions. Parathyroid glands appear as a hypervascular nodule behind the thyroid. In selected patients, multiplanar reconstruction are also obtained [10]. Fig. **4** shows a CT image of an ectopic PT adenoma of the right inferior PT gland.

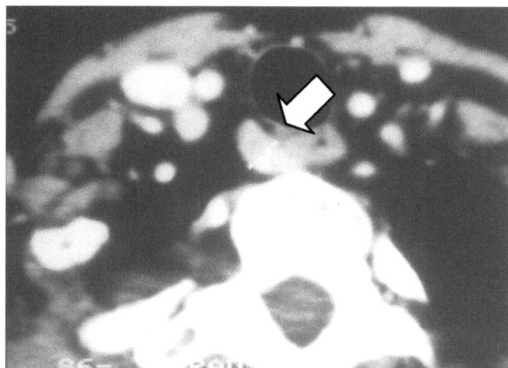

Figure 4: Computed tomography (CT) scanning image showing an ectopic parathyroid adenoma in the right inferior parathyroid gland (arrow) sited in the upper mediastinum, at the retrotracheal space, in a 59-year-old man with primary hyperparathyroidism, who had undergone unsuccessful cervical exploration six months prior to CT.

Magnetic Resonance Imaging

MR study is performed using unenhanced T1- and T2-weighted sequences, as well as contrast-enhanced T1-weighted sequences. MR has long been used in localizing enlarged PT glands, that show a low signal intensity in T1- weighted, and a high signal in T2-weighted sequences (Fig. **5**).

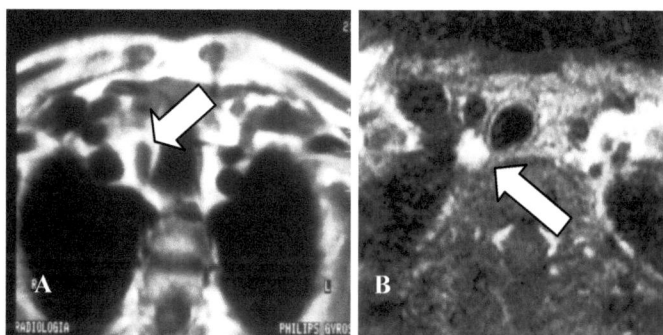

Figure 5: Magnetic resonance imaging in patients with primary hyperparathyroidism. A: T-1 weighted low-intensity signal image showing a parathyroid adenoma on the right aspect of the trachea. B: T-2 weighted image with typical hyperintensity signal at the right of trachea.

Contrast-enhanced T1-weighted sequences obtained after a paramagnetic contrast [gadolinium-diethylene triamine pentaacetic acid (Gd-DTPA)] administration, and fat suppression technique, can be also used [11-13].

Mediastinal PT adenomas can be investigated either with CT scan or MR. They are never in the anterior mediastinum, where only intrathoracic goiters are found, and in the posterior mediastinum, for the embryological reasons described above. More rarely, the PT adenoma is situated within the thyroid gland, usually in a nook excavated on the posterior face of thyroid lobe, mimicking in the CT scan, the appearance of a thyroid tumor. It is not possible to distinguish between thyroid nodule and intrathyroid PT tumor, both on CT and MR imaging. On US, however, a PT tumor is hypoechoic, while a real thyroid nodule located on the posterior face of the thyroid lobe is typically hyperechoic (Fig. **6**).

Ultrasonography

Parathyroids US is usually performed using a 7.5-12 MHz real-time linear transducer, obtaining images from the angle of the mandible to the sternal notch. The typical sonographic appearance of a PT tumor on gray-scale imaging is a nodule nonadherent to the surrounding tissues, oval or oblong in shape, posterior or lateral to the thyroid lobe, ranging from 7 to 20 mm in size [8, 14].

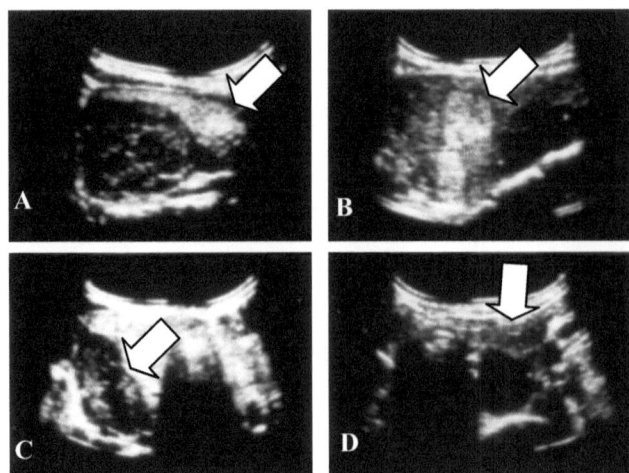

Figure 6: Ultrasonograms of the neck in a patient with primary hyperparathyroidism and multinodular goiter. A & B: Typical hyperechoic thyroid nodule (arrows). C & D: Hypoechoic nodule, suggesting an ectopic parathyroid adenoma localized within the thyroid tissue.

Surgeon-performed US is an emerging, attractive, and accurate technique that facilitates focused and minimally-invasive parathyroidectomy [15]. In experienced hands it may provide cost savings and patient convenience as the first diagnostic procedure for patients suspected to have primary HPT due to a solitary PT adenoma [16]. Endoscopic US and color Doppler US have also been proposed, with the aim of better localizing paraesophageal enlarged PT glands, and to better differentiate PT adenomas from thyroid nodules, respectively [17, 18].

Table **2** reports advantages and disadvantages of US, CT scan and MR imaging in patients with primary HPT.

Table 2: Advantages and disadvantages of US, CT scan, and MR imaging in patients with primary HPT. *retroesophageal, retrotracheal, and deep cervical; PT = parathyroid; PTx = parathyroidectomy; SPECT = ^{99m}Tc sestamibi scintigraphy and single-photon emission computed tomography technique; CT = computed tomography scan; HPT = hyperparathyroidism [21, 22].

Imaging technique	Advantages	Disadvantages
Neck ultrasonography	Easy to perform, no radiation required Sensitive in intrathyroid adenomas	Difficult location of ectopic PT adenomas *
Computed tomography scan	Sensitive in ectopic PT glands Reserved for cases of failed PTx Possibility of performing SPECT/CT	Relatively expensive than US Radiation and contrast required
Magnetic resonance imaging	Good anatomical details, no radiation required, high specificity. Useful in patients with persistent or recurrent HPT	More expensive than US and CT Lower sensitivity than CT scan

Ultrasound-guided fine needle aspiration cytology with or without PTH measurement is useful to confirm the presence of PT tissue, but should be used exclusively in patients scheduled for parathyroidectomy [19, 20].

Parathyroid Scintigraphy

Parathyroid scintigraphy is currently performed using intravenous administration of ^{99m}Tc-methoxyisobutylisonitrile (sestamibi). This radiopharmaceutical, usually used for cardiac function study, was found to be a new agent for PT imaging since 1989 [23]. Its uptake into the hyperfunctioning PT tissue is justified by the presence of a large amount of mithocondria within PT adenomas, together with the absence of p-glycoprotein [24, 25].

The 3 main different sestamibi scan methods are reported in Fig. **7** [21]:

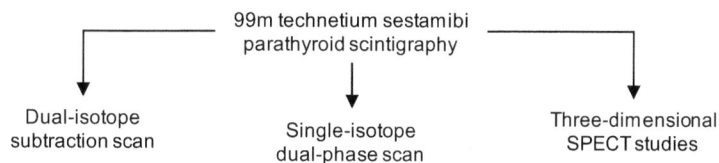

Figure 7: Main different sestamibi scan methods for localizing enlarged parathyroid glands. SPECT = single-photon emission computed tomography.

The single-radionuclide dual-phase study is carried out acquiring images typically 20-30 minutes and two hours after ^{99m}Tc-sestamibi or ^{99m}Tc-tetrofosmin injection. Additional images to localize the thyroid can be obtained using another specific radionuclide, such as ^{99m}Tc-pertechnetate or ^{123}I (dual-isotope scan) [26-28]. Single-photon computed emission tomography (SPECT), and computer reconstruction technique, together with subtraction pinhole images, improve PT-lesion-detection accuracy [28, 29].

In our experience, double-isotope subtraction scan is performed using a single detector gamma camera with a parallel-hole high-resolution collimator [3, 8]. Planar images (head, neck and mediastinum anterior view, matrix 256 × 256) are acquired 5-15 min after intravenous administration of 370 MBq ^{99m}Tc-sestamibi, and thyroid scintigrams are obtained after 150 MBq ^{99m}Tc-pertechnetate injection. A positive result is defined as a relative increasing of sestamibi uptake persisting after image subtraction (Fig. **8**). The sensitivity of sestamibi scintigraphy ranges widely, according to the calcium and PTH serum levels, vitamin D deficiency, size and weight of PT adenomas [3, 30, 31].

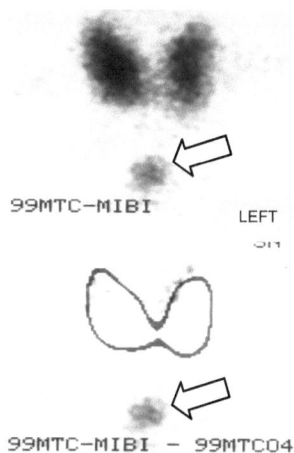

Figure 8: Double-isotope subtraction scintigraphy images in a patients with primary hyperparathyroidism due to a mediastinal parathyroid adenoma.

Top image was acquired 15 min after 370 MBq intravenous administration of ^{99m}Tc-sestamibi, showing both the thyroid gland morphology, and a pathological area of radionuclide uptake in the mediastinum (arrow). Further thyroid scintigrams were obtained after 150 MBq ^{99m}Tc-pertechnetate injection.

A significant extra-tyroidal sestamibi uptake persisting after images subtraction (arrow) confirmed the presence of a non-thyroid tissue in the medistinum, corresponding to a hyperfunctioning ectopic parathyroid gland (Courtesy of F. Bui, MD, and D. Cecchin, MD, Nuclear Medicine Section, University of Padua, Italy).

Other Techniques

When the three-dimensional functional information complemented by sestamibi SPECT-scintigraphy is fused with the anatomic information from CT scan, SPECT/CT images are obtained [32, 33]. This technique is particularly helpful for preoperative localization of ectopic PT adenomas. Four-dimensional CT, and MR and scintigraphy images fusion techniques are also reported [34, 35].

Both ^{18}F-fluoro-2-deoxyglucose (FDG) positron emission tomography (FDG-PET) and 11C-methionine PET have similar sensitivity than sestamibi scintigraphy, as well as PET/CT, but they are very expensive techniques [36, 37]. Selective venous sampling for PTH assay is an invasive, expensive, and technically difficult way to localize hyperfunctioning PT glands. It is obsolete at present, and was used exclusively when negative or non-concordant results of imaging studies were achieved, representing the third-step of the preoperative evaluation of patients with persistent or recurrent HPT [38, 39].

RENAL & BONE IMAGING IN HYPERPARATHYROIDISM

Currently, from 80% to 90% of patients with primary HPT are asymptomatic or minimally symptomatic (see Chapter 2). Kidney stones, usually calcium oxalate stones, occur in about 10% of patients with primary HPT, while only 5% of those with nephrolithiasis may have PT glands hyperfunction and hypercalcemia (see Chapter 1). However, in patients with primary HPT the kidney involvement may be related either to recurrent nephrolithiasis or calcium deposition of calcium in the renal parenchyma. However, renal function impairment leading to polyuria due to the loss of concentrating ability, is observed only in patients with severe and untreated disease. The radiological study of renal stones includes plain abdominal x-ray, US, and unenhanced CT scan, particularly useful to search small calcifications within the renal parenchyma, cortical sites (proximal tubules), pyramids, and distal renal ducts. In several studies ultrasonography is of limited value for detecting renal stones, which is dependent on the side of the kidney involved, with an overall sensitivity of about 50%, and 70-80% accuracy [40, 41]. Unenhanced helical CT has become the primary imaging modality for evaluating acute flank pain and suspected renal stone disease, particularly for detecting ureteral calculi, which often are not visualized with other imaging modalities. Thus, both US and intravenous pyelography have begun to play a secondary role in the evaluation of genitourinary calculi [40, 42].

The classic features of hyperparathyroid bone disease, as well as nephrocalcinosis due to elevated calcium content within the kidneys, are today extremely uncommon in patients with primary HPT, even though they have a long history of complications of the disease (see Chapter 2). Histologically, in bones with o*steitis fibrosa cystica* an increased number of osteoclasts is observed, together with marrow fibrosis and cysts frequently containing fibrous tissue and *foci* of osteoid tissue, that take place in the normal bone (brown tumors). These classic skeletal manifestations of HPT are today seen exclusively in the rare and severe forms with subperiosteal bone resorption [43, 44]. When these skeletal manifestations were more common, x-ray films showed specific radiological signs (Fig. **9**). Bone lesions were especially found in hand fingers and forearms. Moreover, salt-and-pepper appearance of the skull, and a nonspecific loss of the *lamina dura* of the teeth were also observed.

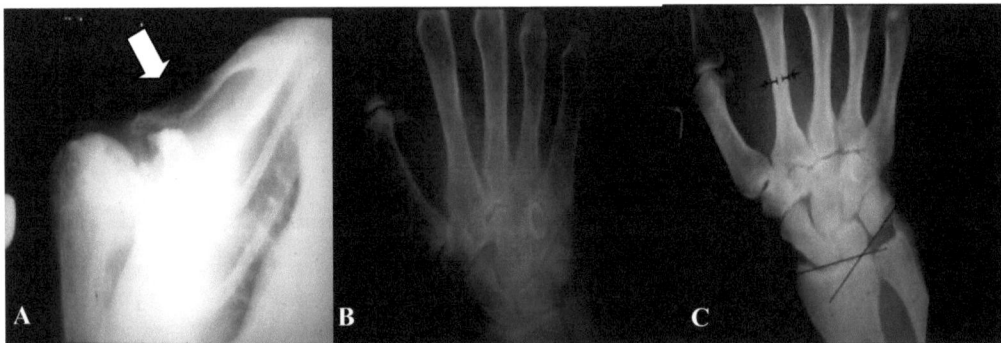

Figure 9: (A) X-ray of shoulder showing a bone defect of the clavicle, corresponding to a pseudocystic mass (arrow) filled with hemorrhagic fluid and fibrous tissue (brown tumor) in a 52-year-old women with severe untreated primary hyperparathyroidism. B: Hand and wrist x-ray from the same patient, demonstrating metacarpal bones osteoporosis, and typical bone cortex reduction, compared to normal carpal bones (C).

Pathological vertebral fractures due to HPT were inclined to repair with bone callus formation, having the so called "black arumband" typical appearance. However, they underwent complete repair once bone mineral balance was restored after surgery.

Brown tumors were usually asymptomatic, causing pain and fractures in undiagnosed patients. On an x-ray they appear as lytic *foci* with tortuous contours and margins well defined, without sclerosis. In isolated cases, CT may disclose a mass that enhances after contrast injection, not involving soft tissues, without periosteal reaction [44].

Direct measurement of bone density (BMD) is usually obtained by either dual-energy x-ray absorptiometry (DXA) or quantitative computed tomography (QCT), that measures trabecular bone density in the spine, both useful in assessing fracture risk and drug efficacy [45]. DXA is a biplanar method that provides a projectional measurement of BMD, and determines areal density at the lumbar spine, hip, and wrist, with the precision error of less than 2% [1]. The World Health Organization has long defined osteoporosis as a BMD > 2.5 standard deviations below the young normal mean (T-score) (see Chapter 2).

Quantitative computed tomography is a volumetric density measurement, for unit of volume at lumbar spine, unaffected by differences in bone size. The advantage over DXA is represented by its ability to specifically measure the trabecular bone mineral content with excellent precision, separating by cortical bone, and it can be obtained in any CT scan made for other reasons, while DXA measures both together [46]. The QCT is evaluated in mg of mineral content/mL of bone of the spongious vertebral one.

MALIGNANCY-ASSOCIATED HYPERCALCEMIA

The imaging study of patients with malignancy-associated hypercalcemia (MAH) is required when the primary tumor leading to hypercalcemia is unknown. There are two main causes of MAH: (1) osteolytic (i.e. bone metastases from lung, breast, prostate, thyroid and renal cancer), and more frequently (2) humoral, due to a paraneoplastic syndrome in which increased parathyroid hormone-related protein (PTHrP) serum levels causes osteoclast activation, and subsequent calcium reasbsorption (see Chapter 3).

Myeloma and metastatic squamous cell carcinoma of the lung account for more than 50% of cases of MAH [47]. The imaging studies useful in patients with MAH are reported in Fig. **10**.

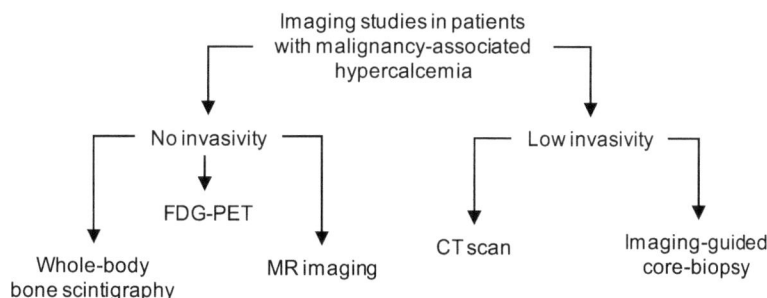

Figure 10: Imaging studies in patients with malignancy-associated hypercalcemia. FDG-PET=[18F]-2-fluorodeoxyglucose positron emission tomography, MR=magnetic resonance, CT=computed tomography.

Skeletal metastases are a major clinical problem for the oncologist. They significantly affect prognosis and may result in pathologic fractures, neurologic impairment, as well as hypercalcemia and bone pain [48]. In case of suspected malignancy, a multimodality approach is needed for a whole-bone assessment. The study includes plain radiograms (x-ray), whole-body bone scintigraphy (WBS), CT scan, and MR imaging, while FDG-PET and PET-CT are considered as second-level study. Bone x-rays are used as a basic imaging procedure or to analyze a painful area, while CT scan is considered the method of choice in the assessment of bone stability and risk of fracture [49]. Fig. **11** reports a suggested algorithm for bone metastases detection.

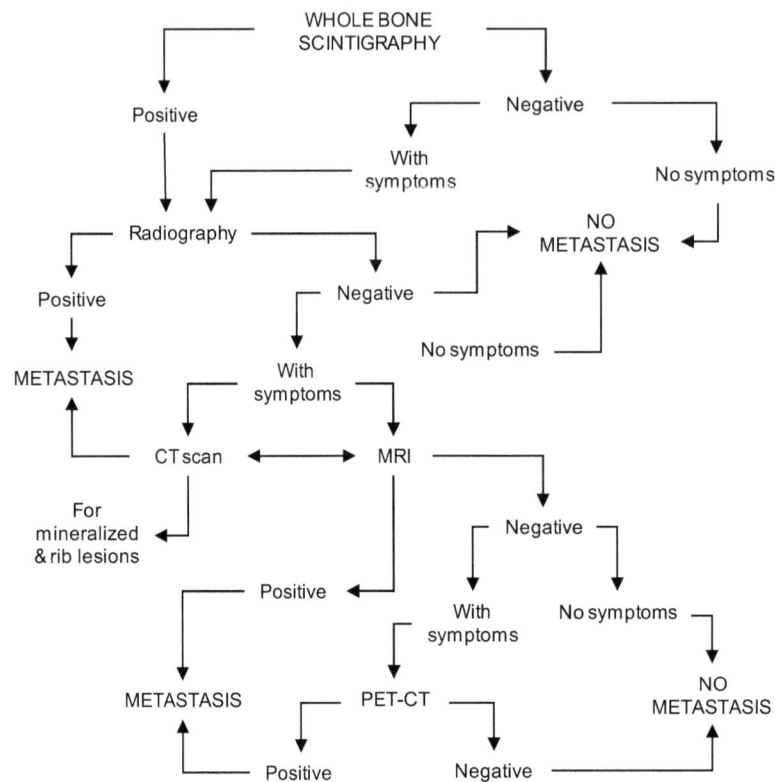

Figure 11: Possible algorithm for detection of metastatic bone disease. CT = computed tomography scan, MRI = magnetic resonance imaging, PET-CT = [18F]-2-fluorodeoxyglucose positron emission tomography-CT. Modified from [50] and [52].

Whole-Body Bone Scintigraphy

Bone scan has a pivotal role in the detection of skeletal bone disease, visualizing increases in osteoblastic activity and skeletal vascularity [51]. It is used extensively, and offers the advantage of total body examination, showing bone lesions earlier than other techniques. In case of clinical suspicion, such as pain or serum tumor markers elevation, it should be used as the first step imaging technique, because of its high sensitivity and low cost [52-54].

Bone scan is usually performed using 99m-technetium labeled bisphosphonates (^{99m}Tc-MDP) administration. Its sensitivity ranges between 70-100%, and specificity between 80-100%. Although WBS is more sensitive than x-rays, it should be considered a screening imaging technique because it detects all aspecific metabolic bone reaction, including posttraumatic lesions and other benign diseases. On the other hand, a pathological decrease of 30-75% in mineral bone content is needed to be detected by x-rays [55, 56].

For these reasons, the SPECT technique has been proposed to increase sensitivity, resulting especially useful in the evaluation of complex areas, such as pelvis and spine, and to rule out "hot spots" found at standard WBS, resulting more accurate than FDG-PET in the detection of sclerotic metastases [57, 58].

Magnetic Resonance Imaging and CT Scan

Since WBS reveals only bone metabolism, an appropriate imaging technique should follow the first approach. Both MR imaging and CT scan can depict anatomic changes better than WBS. It has long been established that CT is able to differentiate bone density with high detail (using appropriate window), and well delineate bone cortex. It may characterize abnormal calcifications and it is useful in confirming bone disease, because it is able to show all bone components and contiguous bone tissues

[59]. CT scan is preferable to MR imaging in the assessment of cortex, rib's disease, and evaluation of the possible risk of fractures. Differently, MR imaging has an excellent soft-tissue resolution, and is preferable in evaluation of bone marrow and spinal disease, differentiating between osteoporotic and malignant vertebral fractures, but is less effective in the evaluation bone loss tissue [60]. Although CT scan and MR imaging have a different sensitivity, the latter allows a direct visualization of bone marrow components, with high spatial resolution.

The unique soft-tissue contrast of MR enables precise assessment of bone marrow infiltration, before osteolytic changes become visible on CT, and metabolic changes occur in WBS and PET [60]. The use of paramagnetic contrast increases the accuracy in differentiating necrotic tissue and evaluating response to therapy [52]. Very recently, advances in technology have made high resolution whole-body MR imaging (WB-MRI) clinically feasible. WB-MRI is expensive, but has many advantages, such as absence of ionizing radiation and high accuracy for detection of skeletal metastases and staging of hematological disease [60]. WB-MRI has also found to be more effective than WBS in the detection of bone metastases, and more sensitive then PET-CT [50].

Positron Emission Tomography

PET detects the uptake of positron-emitting radiopharmaceuticals. [^{18}F]-fluoro-2-deoxyglucose is used because of the high glucose uptake of several tumors, and this tumor tracer accumulates in bone tissues, depending on osteoblastic activity and local blood flow. The functional imaging can be combined with a better three-dimension anatomical definition of the pathological FDG uptake using the new-generation PET, which includes an integrated CT scan (PET-CT). Higher doses of radiation are administered to the patients, but higher sensitivity and better soft-tissue evaluation are achieved. Sensitivity of FDG-PET for detection of bone metastases ranges between 70-100%, and specificity between 95-100%. Possible disadvantages are high cost and lack of availability. PET is very promising in assessment of response to treatment of several malignancies, but its usefulness in bone involvement is still debated, because FDG uptake can be increased by chemotherapy [52]. If imaging studies cannot diagnose the origin of a bone mass, imaging-guided core-biopsy should be performed.

OTHER DISEASES CAUSING HYPERCALCEMIA

Multiple Myeloma

Myeloma is a low-grade non-Hodgkin's B-cell lymphoma, characterized by a proliferation of monoclonal malignant plasma cells. It occurs mainly in middle- or advanced-age men. As malignant plasma cells increase in number, they gradually replace normal marrow [61]. Bone involvement is typically multiple, and during the evaluation of the disease, nearly 50% of patients develop bone pain and neurologic symptoms, most often secondary to compression of the spinal cord due to vertebral body compression fractures and/or epidural spread of the disease [62]. Three different patterns can be found at imaging: diffuse bone marrow involvement, focal bone destruction by solid nodules, and extraosseous manifestations [61]. Bone lesions appear as multiple osteolytic areas with variable size and clear limits, usually localized at the spine or ribs. Compact bone is eroded internally, and then destroyed with consequent soft tissue invasion, visible on CT and MR imaging. Classically, any periostial reaction is absent and often, in pelvis and spine, bone lesions mimic osteoporosis [61]. The MRI is the most sensitive technique for detection of myeloma lesions, which are hypointense on T1-weighted images and hyperintense on T2-weighted images, similar to metastasis [63].

Sarcoidosis

Sarcoidosis is a systemic disease of unknown etiology characterized by noncaseating granulomas, and a wide range of radiologic and clinical manifestations. Hypercalcemia may be found in about 20% of cases. Thoracic involvement occurs in 80-90% of patients, who tipically present a symmetric mediastinal and hilar adenopathy on chest x-ray, and CT scan, detecting both the lymphadenopathy and its extent, and parenchymal lung disease [64]. Chest CT can be performed in three basic formats: conventional chest CT, standard high resolution CT (HRCT), and volumetric HRCT. CT features include thoracic lymphoadenopathy, typically bilateral and non-necrotic, nodules and ground glass opacities [65]. On HRCT, small (2 to 3 mm) nodules may be seen within the parenchyma, sometimes accompanied by slightly larger, typically irregular, nodules along the pleura and fissures. Gadolinium-MR imaging has an important role in the early detection of cardiac involvement, which is the main cause of death related to untreated disease [65].

CONCLUSIONS

The imaging studies to approach patients with hypercalcemia can be summarized as following:

- Primary HPT: The first studies should be US and sestamibi scintigraphy. If they are negative or discordant, ectopic PT glands are suspected. Therefore, the CT scan, MRI or more recently PET should be suggested.

- Urinary tract: US has a good accuracy in the detection of renal stones, but unenhanced CT scan has the best sensitivity.

- Bone metastases: The first imaging technique is whole bone scintigraphy, followed by plan x-ray of single sites. CT scan and/or MRI may complete the differential diagnosis. CT scan is suggested for mineralized and rib lesions, while MR is preferable for bone marrow lesions. FDG-PET is useful in detection of soft tissue or bone metastases. In case of unknown origin, an image-guided core-biopsy should be performed.

REFERENCES

[1]   Shoback D, Marcus R, Bikle D, Strewler G. Mineral metabolism & metabolic bone disease. In: Greenspan FS & Gardner DG, Eds. Basic & Clinical Endocrinology. New York, Lange Medical Books/McGraw Hill, 2001; pp. 237-333.

[2]   Bilezikian JP, Khan AA, Potts JT. Guidelines for the management of asymptomatic Primary Hyperparathyroidism: summary statement from the Third International Workshop. J Clin Endocrinol Metab 2009; 94: 335-339.

[3]   Lumachi F, Ermani M, Basso S, *et al.* Localization of parathyroid tumours in the minimally invasive era: which technique should be chosen ? Population-based analysis of 253 patients undergoing parathyroidectomy and factors affecting parathyroid gland detection. Endocr Relat Cancer 2001; 8: 63-69.

[4]   Grant CS, Thompson G, Farley D, van Heerden J. Primary hyperparathyroidism surgical management since the introduction of minimally invasive parathyroidectomy. Mayo Clinic experience. Arch Surg 2005; 140: 472-478.

[5]   Akerström G, Malmaeus J, Bergström R. Surgical anatomy of human parathyroid glands. Surgery 1984: 95: 14-21.

[6]   Herrera MF, Gamboa-Dominguez A. Parathyroid embryology, anatomy, and pathology. In: Clark OH, Duh Q-Y, Kebebew E, Eds. Textbook of Endocrine Surgery. Philadelphia, Elsevier Saunders, 2005; pp. 365-371.

[7]   Lumachi F, Zucchetta P, Varotto S, *et al.* Noninvasive localization procedures in ectopic hyperfunctioning parathyroid tumors. Endocr Relat Cancer 1999; 6: 123-125.

[8]   Lumachi F, Marzola MC, Zucchetta P, Tregnaghi A, Cecchin D, Bui F. Hyperfunctioning parathyroid tumours in patients with thyroid nodules. Sensitivity and positive predictive value of high-resolution ultrasonography and ^{99m}Tc-sestamibi scintigraphy. Endocr Relat Cancer 2003; 10: 419-423.

[9]   Lumachi F, Tregnaghi A, Zuchetta P, *et al.* Technetium-99m sestamibi scintigraphy and helical CT together in patients with primary hyperparathyroidism: a prospective clinical study. Br J Radiol 2004; 77: 100-103.

[10]   Zald PB, Hamilton BE, Larsen ML, Cohen JI. The role of computed tomography for localization of parathyroid adenomas. Laryngoscope 118; 1405-1410.

[11]   Auffermann W, Gooding GA, Okelund MD, *et al.* Diagnosis of recurrent hyperparathyroidism: comparison of MR imaging and the other techiniques. AJR 1988; 150: 1027-1033.

[12]   Auffermann W, Guis M, Traveres NJ, Higgins CB. MR signal intensity of parathyroid adenomas: correlation with histopathology. AJR 1989; 153: 873-876.

[13] Munk RS, Payne RJ, Luria BJ, Hier MP, Black MJ. Preoperative localization in primary hyperparathyroidism. J Otolaryngol Head Neck Surg 2008; 37 :347-354.

[14] Lumachi F, Zucchetta P, Marzola MC, *et al.* Advantages of combined technetium-99m-sestamibi scintigraphy and high-resolution ultrasonography in parathyroid localization: comparative study in 91 patients with primary hyperparathyroidism. Eur J Endocrinol 2000; 143: 755-760.

[15] Solorzano, CC, Lee TM, Ramirez MC, Carneiro DM, Irvin GL. Surgeon-performed ultrasound improves localization on abnormal parathyroid glands. Am Surg 2005; 71: 557-562.

[16] Arora S, Balash PR, Yoo J, Smith GS, Prinz RA. Benefits of surgeon-performed ultrasound for primary hyperparathyroidism. Langenbecks Arch Surg 2009; 394: 861-867.

[17] Catargi B, Raymond JM, Lafarge-Gense V, Leccia F, Roger P, Tabarin A. Localization of parathyroid tumours using endoscopic ultrasonography in primary hyperparathyroidism. J Endocrinol Invest 1999; 22: 688-692.

[18] Gooding GA, Clark OH. Use of color Doppler imaging in the distinction between thyroid and parathyroid lesions. Am J Surg 1992; 164: 51-56.

[19] Kiblut NK, Cussac JF, Soudan B, *et al.* Fine needle aspiration and intraparathyroid intact parathyroid hormone measurement for reoperative parathyroid surgery. World J Surg 2004; 28: 1143-1147.

[20] Maser C, Donovan P, Santos F, *et al.* Udelsman R. Sonographically guided fine needle aspiration with rapid parathyroid hormone assay. Ann Surg Oncol 2006; 13: 1690-1695.

[21] Rodriguez JM, Parilla P. Localization studies in persistent or recurrent hyperparathyroidism. In: Clark OH, Duh Q-Y, Kebebew E, Eds. Textbook of Endocrine Surgery. Philadelphia, Elsevier Saunders, 2005; pp. 430-438.

[22] Shah S, Win Z, Al-Nahhas A. Multimodality imaging of the parathyroid glands in primary hyperparathyroidism. Minerva Endocrinol 2008; 33: 193-202.

[23] Coakley AJ, Kettle AG, Wells CP, O'Doherty MJ, Collins RE. 99m-Technetium sestamibi. A new agent for parathyroid imaging. Nucl Med Commun 1989; 10: 791-794.

[24] Mitchel BK, Cornelius EA, Zoghbi S, *et al.* Mechanism of technetium 99m sestamibi parathyroid imaging and the possible role of the p-glycoprotein. Surgery 1996; 120: 1039-1045

[25] Gupta Y, Ahmed R, Happerfield L, Pinder SE, Balan KK, Wishart GC. P-glycoprotein expression is associated with sestamibi washout in primary hyperparathyroidism. Br J Surg 2007; 94: 1491-1495.

[26] Taillefer R, Boucher Y, Potvin C, Lambert R. Detection and localization of parathyroid adenomas in patients with hyperparathyroidism using a single radionuclide imaging procedure with technetium 99m sestamibi (double-phase study). J Nucl Med 1992; 33: 1801-1807.

[27] Freudemberg LS, Frilling A, Sheu SY, Gorges R. Optimizing operative imaging in primary hyperparathyroidism. Langenbecks Arch Surg 2006; 391: 551-556.

[28] Mihai R, Simon D, Hellman P. Imaging for primary hyperparathyroidism. An evidence-based analysis. Langenbecks Arch Surg 2009; 394: 765-784.

[29] Nichols KJ, Tomas MB, Tronco GG, *et al.* Preoperative parathyroid scintigraphic lesion localization: accuracy of various types of readings. Radiology 2008; 248: 221-232.

[30] Erbil Y, Barbaros U, Yanik BT, *et al.* Impact of gland morphology and concomitant thyroid nodules on operative localization of parathyroid adenomas. Laryngoscope 2006; 116: 580-585.

[31] Kandil E, Tufaro AP, Carrson KA, *et al.* Correlation of plasma 25-hydroxyvitamin D levels with severity of primary hyperparathyroidism and likelihood of parathyroid adenoma localization on sestamibi scan. Arch Otolayngol Head Neck Surg 2008; 134: 1071-1075.

[32] Profanter C, Wetscher GJ, Gabriel M, *et al.* CT-MIBI image fusion: a new preoperative localization technique for primary, recurrent, and persistent hyperparathyroidism. Surgery 2004; 135: 157-162.

[33] Eslamiy HZ, Ziessman HA. Parathyroid scintigraphy in patients with primary hyperparathyroidism: 99mTc sestamibi SPECT and SPECT/CT. Radiographics 2008; 28: 1461-1476.

[34] Rodgers SE, Hunter GJ, Hamberg LM, *et al.* Improved preoperative planning for directed parathyroidectomy with 4-dimensional computed tomography. Surgery 2006; 140: 932-940.

[35] Ruf J, Lopez Hanninen E, Steinmuller T, *et al.* Preoperative localization of parathyroid glands. Use of MRI, scintigraphy, and image fusion. Nuklearmedizin 2004; 43: 85-90.

[36] Beggs AD, Hain SF. Localization of parathyroid adenomas using 11C-methionine positron emission tomography. Nucl Med Commun 2005; 26: 1766-1770.

[37] Tang BN, Moreno-Reyes R, Blocklet D, *et al.* Accurate pre-operative localization of pathological parathyroid glands using 11C-methionine PET/CT. Contrast Media Mol Imaging 2008; 3: 157-163.

[38] Chaffanjon PC, Voirin D, Vasdev A, Chabre O, Kenyon NM, Brichon PY. Selective venous sampling in recurrent and persistent hyperparathyroidism: indication, technique, and results. World J Surg 2000; 28: 958-961.

[39] Eloy JA, Mitty H, Genden EM. Preoperative selective venous sampling for nonlocalizing parathyroid adenomas. Thyroid 2006; 16: 787-790.

[40] Fower KA, Locken JA, Duchesne JH, Williamson MR. US for detecting renal calculi with nonenhanced CT as a reference standard. Radiology 2002; 222: 109-113.

[41] Ulusan S, Koc Z, Tokmak N. Accuracy of sonography for detecting renal stone: comparison with CT. J Clin Ultrasound 2007; 35: 256-261.

[42] Amis ES Jr. Epitaph for the urogram. Radiology 1999; 213:639-640.

[43] Azria A, Beaudreuil J, Juquel JP, Quillard A, Bardin T. Brown tumor of the spine revealing secondary hyperparathyroidism. Report of a case. Joint Bone Spine 2000; 67: 230-233.

[44] Jouan A, Zabraniecki L, Vincent V, Poix E, Fournié B. An unusual presentation of primary hyperparathyroidism: severe hypercalcemia and multiple brown tumors. Report of a case. Joint Bone Spine 2008; 75: 209-211.

[45] Leib ES, Lenchik L, Bilezikian JP, Mericic MJ, Watts NB. Position statements of the International Society for Clinical Densitometry: methodology. J Clin Densitom 2002; 5: S5-S10.

[46] Link TM, Majumdar S. Osteoporosis imaging. Radiol Clin North Am 2003; 41: 813-839.

[47] Lumachi F, Brunello A, Roma A, Basso U. Cancer-induced hypercalcemia. Anticancer Res 2009; 29: 1551-1556.

[48] Brown SA, Guise TA. Cancer treatment-related bone disease. Crit Rev Eukaryot Gene Expr 2009; 19: 47-60.

[49] Schmidt GP, Reiser MF, Baur-Melnyk A. Whole-body imaging of bone marrow. Semin Musculoskelet Radiol. 2009; 13:120-33.

[50] Costelloe CA, Rohren EM, Madewell JE, *et al.* Imaging bone metastases in breast cancer: technique and recommendations for diagnosis. Lancet Oncol 2009; 10: 606-614.

[51] Krasnow AZ, Hellman RS, Timins ME, Collier BD, Anderson T, Isitman AT. Diagnostic bone scanning in oncology. Semin Nucl Med 1997; 27: 107-141.

[52] Hamaoka T, Madewell JE, Podoloff DA, Hortobagyi GN, Ueno NT. Bone imaging in metastatic breast cancer. J Clin Oncol 2004; 22: 2942-2953.

[53] Lumachi F, Brandes AA, Ermani M, Bruno G, Boccagni P. Sensitivity of serum tumor markers CEA and CA 15-3 in breast cancer recurrences and correlation with different prognostic factors. Anticancer Res 2000; 20: 4751-4756.

[54] Lumachi F, Basso SMM, Basso U. Breast cancer recurrence: role of serum tumor markers CEA and CA 15-3. In: Hayat MA, Ed. Methods of Cancer Diagnosis, Therapy, and Prognosis. Volume 1, Breast Carcinoma. Heidelberg, Springer Science, 2008; pp. 109-115.

[55] Vinholes J, Coleman R, Eastell R. Effects of bone metastases on bone metabolism: implications for diagnosis, imaging and assessment of response to cancer treatment. Cancer Treat Rev 1996; 22: 289-331.

[56] Rybak LD, Rosenthal DI. Radiological imaging for the diagnosis of bone metastases. Q J Nucl Med 2001; 45: 53-64.

[57] Savelli G, Maffioli L, Maccauro M, De Deckere E, Bombardieri E. Bone scintigraphy and the added value of SPECT (single photon emission tomography) in detecting skeletal lesions. Q J Nucl Med. 2001;45:27-37.

[58] Uematsu T, Yuen S, Yukisawa S, *et al.* Comparison of FDG-PET and SPECT for detection of bone metastases in breast cancer. Am J Roentgenol 2005; 184: 1266-1273.

[59] Zimmer WD, Berquist TH, McLeod RA, *et al.* Bone tumors: magnetic resonance imaging versus computed tomography. Radiology 1985; 155: 709-718.

[60] Schmidt GP, Reiser MF, Baur-Melnyk A. Whole-body MRI for the staging and follow-up of patients with metastasis. Eur J Radiol 2009; 70: 393-400.

[61] Delorme S, Baur-Melnyk A. Imaging in multiple myeloma. Eur J Radiol 2009; 70: 401-408.

[62] Van Goethem JW, van den Hauwe L, Ozsarlak O, et al. Spinal tumors. Eur J Radiol 2004;50:159-176.

[63] Rahmouni A, Divine K, Mathieu D, *et al.* Detection of multiple myeloma involving the spine: efficacy of fat-suppression and contrast-enhanced MR imaging. AJR 1993;160: 1049-1052.

[64] Hamper UK, Fishman EK, Khouri NF, *et al*. Typical and atypical CT manifestations of pulmonary sarcoidosis. J Comput Assist Tomogr 1986; 10: 928-936.

[65] Akbar JJ, Meyer CA, Shipley RT, Vagal AS. Cardiopulmonary imaging in sarcoidosis. Clin Chest Med 2008; 29: 429-443.

CHAPTER 7

Surgical Treatment of Hypercalcemia

Stefano M.M. Basso[1] and Franco Lumachi[2]

[1]Division of Surgery I, S. Maria degli Angeli Hospital, 33170 Pordenone, Italy and [2]University of Padua, School of Medicine, 35128 Padova, Italy

Abstract: In patients with hypercalcemia the surgical treatment is likely limited to those with primary hyperparathyroidism (HPT), which represents the most frequent cause of this biochemical alteration. Hypercalcemia may also occur in up to 30% of patients with cancer, but unfortunately they are usually unsuitable for surgery. Surgery of parathyroid glands is particularly challenging, because PT anatomy is one of the variables of our organism. The treatment of choice for patients with symptomatic primary HPT is removal of the affected parathyroid(s), that can be achieved both by surgical and non-surgical techniques. The latter is used only in selected patients, when surgery is contraindicated. In asymptomatic patients, surgical parathyroidectomy is usually suggested to prevent complications, but its role is controversial. Bilateral cervical exploration has been the procedure of choice for decades, and it is still mandatory in case of suspicion of multiglandular disease or malignancy, and multiple endocrine neoplasia or familial syndromes. Recent advances in preoperative localization studies, and intraoperative adjuncts, such as quick parathyroid hormone assay, encouraged as a less invasive surgery. Currently, minimally invasive parathyroidectomy is widely performed, both videoassisted and radioguided. Considering the significant improvements of clinical features of the disease after surgery, and the effectiveness and safety of minimally invasive surgical techniques, parathyroidectomy should be suggested both in symptomatic patients and in those with minimally symptomatic primary HPT. However, each patient should be referred to an experienced parathyroid surgeon or endocrinologist, with the aim of having a better definition of the disease, and the best recommendation for treatment.

INTRODUCTION

In patients with hypercalcemia the surgical treatment is likely limited to those with primary hyperparathyroidism (HPT), which represents the most frequent cause of this biochemical alteration. All patients with symptomatic confirmed primary HPT should undergo surgery, with a recovery rate of 95%-98% of the cases when the operation is performed by experienced surgeons.

Hypercalcemia may also occur in up to 30% of patients with a variety of malignant or, less frequently, benign tumors [1, 2]. This severe paraneoplastic syndrome, known as malignancy-associated hypercalcemia (MAH), is related to different types of cancer, such as lung and breast carcinoma, and multiple myeloma [3, 4]. It represents usually the late stage of a metastatic disease, and thus these patients are usually unsuitable for surgery (see Chapter 3). Their prognosis is poor, but the steadily and rapidly progressive hypercalcemia, usually requires rehydration and bisphosphonates administration (see Chapters 4 and 8).

Other causes of hypercalcemia, such as granulomatous diseases and endocrine diseases, should be carefully excluded, and treated by specific drugs (see Chapter 2).

HISTORY OF THE PARATHYROID GLANDS

The history of parathyroid (PT) glands is fascinating and covers the last two centuries. They were identified in 1850 by Sir Richard Owen in the Indian rhinoceros. Viktor Ivar Sandström, a Swedish medical student, named these small glands *glandulae parathyroideae*, when he first identified the parathyroids in humans in 1877 [5]. Unfortunately, the importance of this discovery was initially neglected.

Hypocalcemic tetany, described in 1879 by Anton Wölfer after total thyroidectomy performed by Christian Theodor Billroth, was not associated to concomitant parathyroidectomy (PTx). These patients were considered curiosities, and this sign inexplicable. In 1904 Max Askanazy, a German pathologist, presented the case of *osteitis fibrosa cystica* in a patient with a parathyroid tumor, but missed the relationship between the diseases [6]. In 1906, the anatomist Jakob Erdheim associated PT enlargement and osteomalacia, but only Friedrick Schlagenhaufer in 1915 hypothesized that PT disease was the cause of bone disease, and not the result.

The first successful PTx was performed in Vienna by Felix Mandl in 1925, and in the next decade more than 100 cases of HPT were reported by surgeons such as Emil Theodor Kocher and Williams S. Halsted, who began to write the history of this surgery [7]. Concomitant advances in biochemical and pathophysiological findings encouraged the progress in this field.

ANATOMY OF THE PARATHYROID GLANDS

Surgery of PT glands is particularly challenging, because PT anatomy is one of the variables of our organism. Parathyroid means "beside the thyroid", which is the typical location of these glands, at the posterior surface of the lateral lobes of the thyroid, or close to their inferior border (Fig. 1).

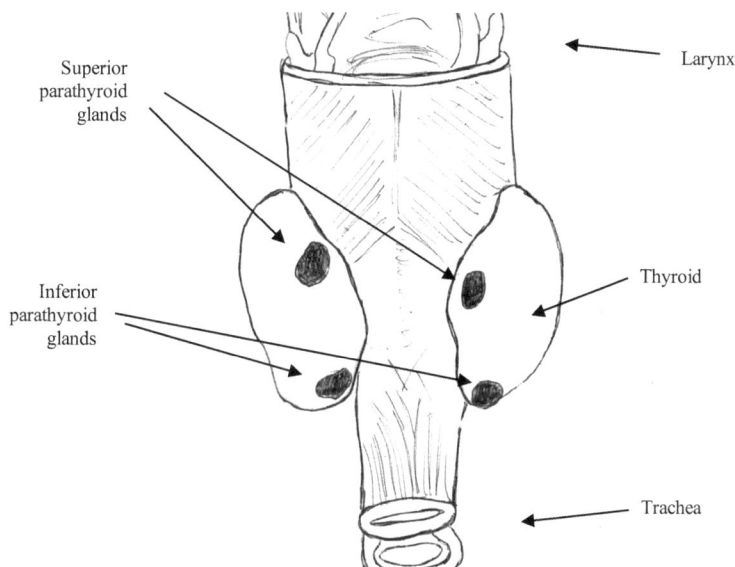

Figure 1: Schematic representation of normal location of the parathyroid glands (posterior view).

The microscopic structure of the PT glands differs from that of the thyroid, since they have densely packed cells in contrast with the follicular cells of varying size of the thyroid. However, at surgery it may be difficult to differentiate normal PT glands from small thyroid nodules or fat. Normally, the glands weigh 25-40 mg each (>60 mg is considered abnormal), and their size ranges from 4 mm to 6 mm in the largest dimension. Their color has been described as "reddish brown" or "mustard yellow" [8]. Histologically, they are made of two main type of cells: chief cells, which are the most important calcium-sensing cells in the body, and oxyphil cells, both containing parathyroid hormone (PTH) but with different secretory regulation.

Parathyroid glands arise from the interaction of neural crest mesenchyme and third and fourth branchial pouch endoderm. Thus, they have a complex development, early in the embryonegenesis of the neck, and they migrate from a part to another of the neck [9]. The superior glands derive from the fourth pharyngeal pouch, together with thyroid. Because of their relatively circumscribed migration, their position in adults is quite constant, being usually located close to the posterolateral side of the thyroid lobe, posteromedially to the recurrent laryngeal nerve. In most cases, they can be found at the cricothyroid junction, 1 cm cranially to the intersection between the recurrent laryngeal nerve and the inferior thyroid artery. The inferior glands develop from the third pharyngeal pouch, together with the thymus, having a more variable position than the superior ones. In fact, both thyroid and thymus migrate from the upper into the lower neck and upper chest, "carrying" the PT. Inferior glands are usually found along the thyrothymic ligament, at the lower pole of the thyroid, anterior to the recurrent laryngeal nerve and below the inferior thyroid artery. However, the location of inferior PT glands varies widely, and this is a very important knowledge for a parathyroid surgeon [8, 10]. They may be found from just beneath the mandible to the pericardium, anterior to the carotid artery bifurcation. (Fig. **2**). In 1984 Åkerström and coworkers reported an autopsy study of 503 cases, showing that there are four glands in 84%, three in 3%, and suprannumerary glands in 13% of the cases [8, 11]. The presence of an adenoma in a fifth PT is considered the most common cause of failed neck exploration for primary HPT performed by a skilled surgeon. About 25% of enlarged glands are ectopic, especially the inferior glands that are found within the thymus. In familial HPT, particularly in multiple endocrine neoplasia (MEN), recurrent HPT is relatively frequent even after subtotal PTx. For this reason, in these cases, a transcervical thymectomy should be always performed to remove a possible supernumerary gland [12].

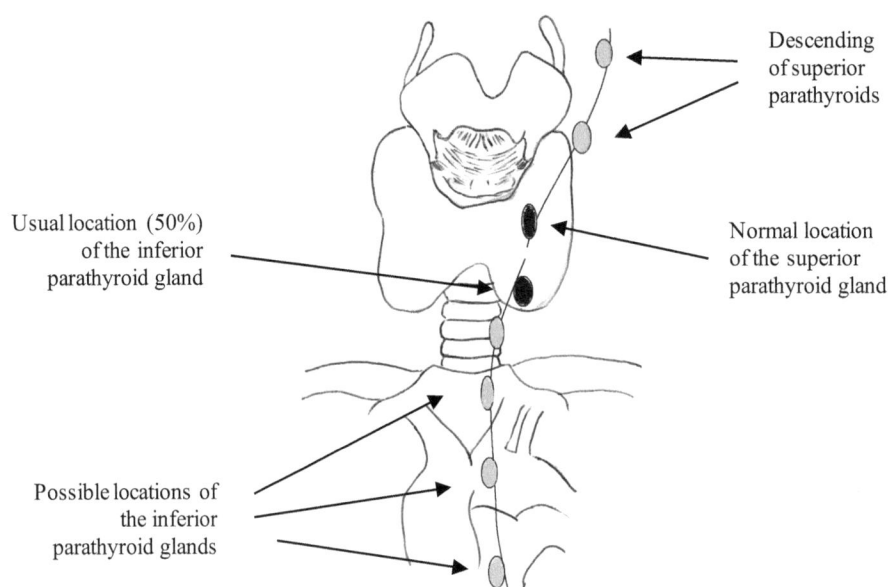

Figure 2: Schematic representation of possible location of the parathyroid glands.

The knowledge of surgical anatomy of the recurrent laryngeal nerve (RLN), which is the motor nerve to the intrinsic muscle of the larynx, represents one of the keys to successful PTx. It is usually accompanied by the inferior laryngeal artery, embedded in the Berry's ligament. The rate of RLN injury, mostly transient, varies from 0.5% to 5% of cases, but increases in reoperative surgery. Abnormalities in the course of RLN is relatively frequent, and thus it should be identified distally, near the cricothyroid joint or just posterior to it, where the anatomy is more constant (Fig. **3**). The RLN originates from the vagus nerve, ascends towards the tracheoesophageal groove, crosses the inferior thyroid artery and the omolateral thyroid lobe, reaching both sides of the larynx. Recent reviews in large series suggest firstly to identify the inferior thyroid artery, and then carefully look for the proximal tract of the nerve [13].

SURGICAL TREATMENT OF PRIMARY HYPERPARATHYROIDISM

Patients with symptomatic HPT usually undergo surgery, while those with asymptomatic HPT are selected according to the guidelines reported in Table **11**. Parathyroidectomy is sometimes required also in patients with secondary HPT. Tertiary HPT, in which PTx is mandatory, is characterized by a lack of suppression of PTH by increasing calcium or vitamin D analogues, usually representing the outcome of longstanding secondary HPT [14].

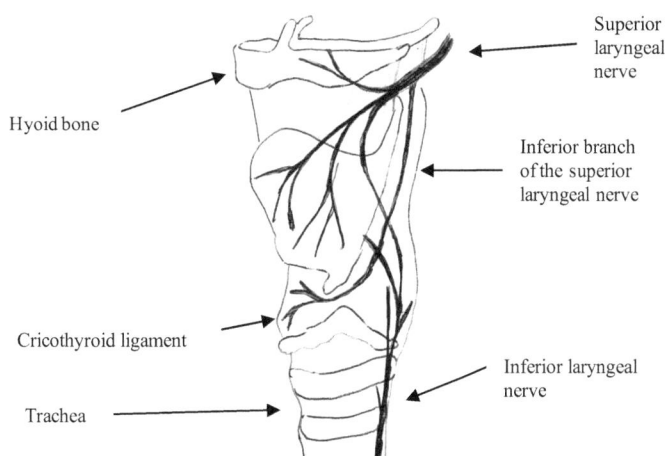

Figure 3: Schematic course of the laryngeal nerves.

The treatment of choice for patients with symptomatic primary HPT is removal of the affected parathyroid(s), that can be achieved both by surgical and non-surgical techniques. The latter is used only in selected patients, when surgery is contraindicated [16]. Table **1** reports possible ablative therapies for primary HPT.

Table 1: Ablative therapies for primary hyperparathyroidism.

Surgical Techniques	Non-surgical Techniques
Bilateral neck exploration	Percutaneous ethanol injection
Unilateral neck exploration	Transcatheter ablation
Selective PTx	Percutaneous laser photocoagulation
Radioguided selective PTx	Percutaneous US-guided radiofrequency
Minimally invasive PTx: - Open PTx with a minimal access - Video-assisted - Endoscopic with or without gas insufflation	
Mediastinal exploration: - Open (cervicotomy, sternotomy, thoracotomy) - Endoscopic (mediastinoscopy or thoracoscopy)	

PTx=parathyroidectomy, US=ultrasound

Among non-surgical techniques, ultrasound-guided percutaneous ethanol injection has been reported to be effective in patients with high surgical risk, advanced disease with severe hypercalcemia, and persistent primary HPT after surgery [15]. In limited series, normalization of both serum calcium and PTH at a 5-year follow-up was obtained in up to 60% of patients, and some clinicians consider it a possible alternative to surgery [17].

Transcatheter ablation of PT adenomas using necrotizing agents, such as ethanol and ionic contrast medium, was shown to be effective only in selected cases, particularly in patients with mediastinal PT adenomas, to avoid sternotomy [18, 19].

In the past, the standard surgical strategy for treating primary HPT was bilateral neck exploration (BNE) necessary to identify each PT gland, fearing of multiple disease [14]. In a retrospective report of 866 BNE performed between 1960 and 1997, a single adenoma and four-gland hyperplasia were found in 77.2% and 21.0% of cases, respectively, with an overall recovery rate of 98.2% after initial cervical exploration [20].

Exploration of the whole neck, followed by the intraoperative identification and excision of the enlarged parathyroid gland(s), was considered the best strategy. When the removed tissue has been confirmed to be a PT adenoma on frozen sections, other specimens should be obtained, to exclude a multiglandular disease [21]. This approach gave good results (>90% of cure), and a very low (1%) morbidity in the hands of experienced surgeons, as reported in several studies in the early 80s [22].

The concept of unilateral neck exploration (UNE) was first suggested by C.A. Wang in the 70s, but applied only in 1982 by S. Tibblin, who started a new era for the PT surgery [23, 24]. This approach was controversial, until other technological advances were introduced. Indeed, accurate preoperative techniques and reliable laboratory tests encouraged remarkable changes in parathyroid surgery during the last two decades [25].

Accurate preoperative localization studies, such as neck ultrasonography (US), sestamibi scintigraphy (MIBI), neck and chest computed tomography scanning (CT) or magnetic resonance imaging (MRI), together with the development of intraoperative quick PTH assay technology (qPTH), explained the trend towards a new and less invasive surgical approach to the PT glands [26].

Minimally invasive PTx have been proposed since 1996, with the aim of reducing operative time, obtaining early discharge of patients and better cosmetic results [27, 28]. However, changes in the surgical strategy are always slow. In fact, in 1991 Kaplan and co-workers stated that "the use of bilateral neck exploration with careful, judicious use of parathyroid biopsy of only one normal appearing gland when an adenoma is present, greatly decreases the chance of missing asymmetric hyperplasia or double adenomas, and gives superior results" [29].

Even if the cost effectiveness of imaging studies is controversial, it has been shown that the concordance between MIBI and US predicts a high chance of recovery, while negative localization studies are highly predictive of multiglandular disease in at least a third of patients with sporadic primary HPT [30]. Furthermore, the former has a better outcome after surgery [31]. Systematic reviews showed that MIBI has a sensitivity ranging from 20% to 95% (median 82%), and US from 25% to 90% (median 82%), confirming that concordant results lead to a positive predictive value (PPV) close to 100% [32, 33]. Thus, the use of at least a preoperative imaging study, followed by intraoperative qPTH assay has been suggested in all patients with primary HPT [34].

Focused approaches have certainly many advantages, but some disadvantages. Some preoparative studies (i.e. MIBI, CT scan) require exposure to radiation (about a half dose of an abdominal CT). However, minimally invasive PTx (MIP) allows smaller access, reduced operative time, lower risk of RLN injury, shorter hospital stay and lower cost [35]. However, a recent study failed to confirm clear clinical advantages and cost-effectiveness of MIP *versus* BNE, being the main clinical objectives (normocalcemia, absence of nerve injuries) similar in both groups [36].

Currently, there is a clear trend towards selective PTx, performed by more than half of the surgeons, even if BNE has still some indications (Fig. **4**). Conversions from MIP are due to: (1) technical difficulties, (2) failure in PT detection, and (3) inadequate post-excision reduction of qPTH. Operations in high-volume centers (>20 cases/year) have a better outcome and less persistent HPT rate [37]. Inexperienced surgeon may fail in detecting abnormal glands, and missed PT glands are found in typical sites at reoperation in up to 80% of cases.

If reoperation is needed, BNE is no longer considered essential. Second-level imaging studies are usually requested (i.e. CT scan and MRI), together with a new biochemical evaluation of the patient, while invasive localization techniques, such as selective venous sampling, should be used only in case of equivocal results of new imaging studies [38]. Recent reviews stated that, if localization studies are significant, a targeted PTx in the neck or chest is still possible, while a careful assessment of vocal cord mobility to exclude a RLN palsy is always recommended [39]. Fig. **5** shows the typical appearance of a PT adenoma.

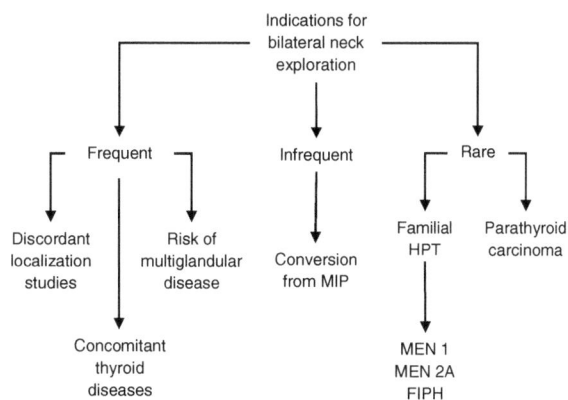

Figure 4: Indications for bilateral neck exploration. MIP = minimally invasive parathyroidec-tomy, HPR = hyperparathyroidism, MEN = multiple endocrine neoplasia, FIPH = familial isolated primary hyperparathyroidism.

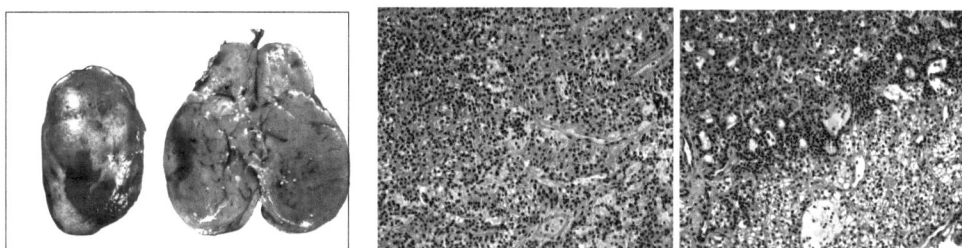

Figure 5: Gross appearance of a parathyroid adenoma (left). Microscopically, it is hypercellular, homogeneous, and well vascularized (center), or composed of an admixture of chief cells and oncocytic cells (right). Original magnification × 400. (Courtesy of F. Marino, MD, Department of Pathology, University of Padua, Italy).

Nowadays, in patients with confirmed primary HPT, MIP should be considered the procedure of choice, especially when preoperative imaging suggest a single PT adenoma [10, 40, 41]. Minimally invasive PTx is performed by 95% of surgeons and, 92% currently use a small-incision technique, either central or lateral [26]. Moreover, in the last years, several alternative approaches have been proposed, in order to avoid any scar in the neck area, such as bilateral axillo-breast incision, and more recently even a postauricolar and axillary endoscopic approach, exclusively for better cosmetic results [42].

Undoubtedly, MIP has several advantages, and the use of videoassisted endoscopic techniques allows a better recognition of the anatomy, through a magnified view and optimal lightning [36, 37]. A number of minimally invasive procedures and acronyms have been reported, such as MIVAP (minimally invasive videoscopically assisted parathyroidectomy), EAMIP (endoscopically assisted minimally invasive parathyroidectomy), and MIRP (minimally invasive radioguided parathyroidectomy). These different approaches to the PT glands, together with the relatively small number of cases, contribute to the lack of evidence-based recommendations, based only on single-center trials, and does not seem to decrease the rate of RLN injury [43, 44].

In 1998 a national survey of USA endocrine surgeons, who were very willing to operate on minimally symptomatic or asymptomatic patients, showed a large divergence in surgical practice and widespread failure to apply the 1990 NIH guidelines, which were updated in 2002 and 2009 [14, 45] (see Chapter 1). Currently, the subgroup of asymptomatic patients with primary HPT accounts for at least 85% of patients, and they might not benefit from surgery.

The result of each type of MIP mainly depends on both preoperative imaging studies sensitivity, and qPTH measurement availability. A recent review concluded that the qPTH assay is not required when a BNE is chosen, and in unilateral explorations in patients with positive MIBI. For MIP with concordant MIBI and US, qPTH is of little value [46]. An analysis of the Scandinavian Register for Thyroid and

Parathyroid Surgery (SRTPS) showed that qPTH correctly confirmed curative surgery in 93.4% of patients, giving 2% false positive and in 4.4% false negative results. In this study, the use of qPTH *versus* no use, increased the rate from 92.3% to 95% [47]. Minimally invasive radioguided parathyroidectomy (MIRP), represents an effective tool for localizing intraoperatively PT adenomas. A positive MIBI scan prior to surgery is required. Presence of thyroid nodules or goiter, risk of multiglandular disease, familial HPT, and lack of concordance between MIBI and US are still considered relative contraindications. Unfortunately, a variety of protocols, isotope dose, and scan sequences are applied in the different centers, and thus there is no clear evidence that MIRP is superior than other techniques, in terms of cost, overall operative time, and length of hospital stay.

To perform MIRP patients should undergo both MIBI and neck US prior to surgery. In the operating room they receive an intravenous injection of 370 MBq ^{99m}Tc-methoxiisobutylisonitrile (sestamibi), 90-120 minutes before the operation was scheduled to start. Four early images are obtained 5 minutes after sestamibi administration. Another technique consists in administrating 50-70 MBq sestamibi 20-30 minutes prior to surgery. In both cases, intraoperative nuclear mapping using a hand-held 11 mm gamma probe is obtained, and quantitative gamma camera counting in the four quadrants is performed. A 2-3 cm incision is made two finger-breadths above the sterna notch, and the adenoma excision is guided by the probe. Removal of the parathyroid adenoma results in a decline in radioactivity in the corresponding quadrant. Finally, the probe is directed away from the patient, and the radioactivity of the removed parathyroid gland is measured and compared with the residual radioactivity obtained scanning the thyroid gland. Intraoperative qPTH assay should be routinely used [14].

Methylen blue dye infusion has been used in the past to better identify intraoperatively enlarged PT glands, but it may cause severe neurological complications. Currently, the routine use of the frozen section examination is not recommended, because misinterpretation of specimens is well known, while qPTH assay of tissue aspirate, in order to discriminate between parathyroid and non-parathyroid tissue, is considered a reliable option [47, 48].

In conclusion, the management of patient with primary HPT is not yet standardized, and an accurate evaluation of each single case is needed. Fig. **6** shows our suggested algorithm in the management of patients with primary HPT.

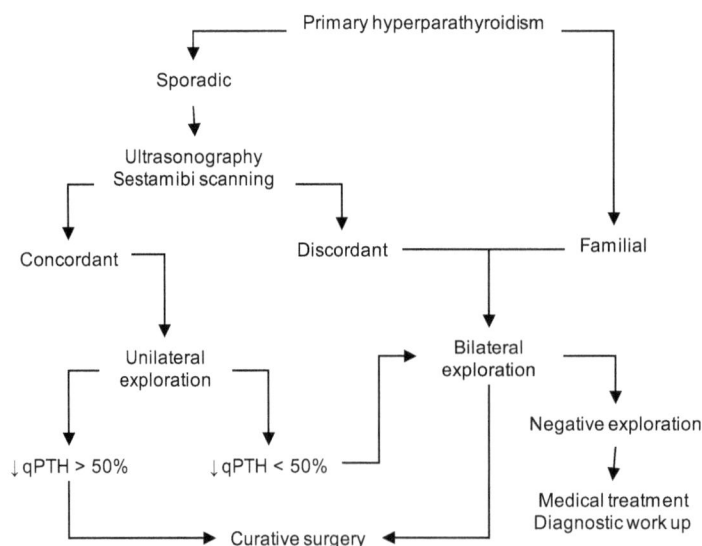

Figure 6: Possible algorithm for the management of patients with symptomatic primary hyperparathyroidism. Successful parathyroidectomy is confirmed when the parathyroid hormone (PTH) falls by 50% or more from baseline, 10-15 minutes following complete resection of parathyroid adenoma. qPTH = intraoperative quick PTH assay (see Chapter 5).

Another cause of hypercalcemia suitable for surgery is PT carcinoma, an uncommon malignancy accounting for 1-2% of cases of primary HPT (see Chapter 2). Natural history and prognostic factors of PT carcinoma are still unclear, and not yet well defined because of the rarity of the disease, while several risk factors, such as the onset in patients with familial hyperparathyroidism-jaw tumor syndrome and MEN syndromes, and the loss of the tumor-suppressor p53 and retinoblastoma (RB) genes have been reported, all accounting for its aggressiveness [49-52]. Clinical presentation (symptomatic bone and renal disease), biochemical finding (severe hypercalcemia and very high serum PTH levels), imaging studies (large PT mass), and intra-operative appearance (tumor strictly adherent to surrounding structures) should address the diagnosis [53, 54].

Another cause of hypercalcemia suitable for surgery is PT carcinoma, an uncommon malignancy accounting for 1-2% of the cases of primary HPT (see Chapter 2). Natural history and prognostic factors of PT carcinoma are still unclear, and not yet well defined because of the rarity of the disease, while several risk factors, such as the onset in patients with familial hyperparathyroidism-jaw tumor syndrome and MEN syndromes, and loss of the tumor-suppressor p53 and retinoblastoma (RB) genes have been reported, all accounting for its aggressiveness [49-52]. Clinical presentation (symptomatic bone and renal disease), biochemical finding (severe hypercalcemia and very high serum PTH levels), imaging studies (large PT mass), and intra-operative appearance (tumor strictly adherent to surrounding structures) should address the diagnosis [53, 54].

Surgery is the only effective treatment for PT carcinoma, and *en-bloc* resection of the tumor and involved peritumoral structures is the recommended primary approach. This usually includes thyroid lobectomy, transcervical thymectomy, and excision of the strap muscle and adjacent soft tissues [53]. Although PT cancer may have an indolent course, recurrence is frequent (50% from 1 to 5 years after initial surgery) and about 25% of patients develop lung and bone metastases during follow-up [54]. The role of adjuvant therapies is still debated, but some retrospective data report a possible benefit from post-operative irradiation [55]. Repeated surgery for recurrence is considered a good palliation to control hypercalcemia, but seems to become less effective when iterative [56]. Severe hypercalcemia, that is ultimately the most frequent cause of death, requires an adequate medical treatment (see Chapter 4).

Secondary HPT is related to hypocalcemia and hyperphosphatemia, common result of chronic renal failure. Its pathogenesis is complex, and a combination of factors contribute to the increase of PTH (see Chapter 1). The chronic long-term stimulation of PT glands cause four-gland hyperplasia, and increases the risk of developing a severe bone disease, leading to *osteitis fibrosa cystica*. Improved medical treatment has decreased the need of PTx in these patients. Cinacalcet, a calcimimetic agent which increases the sensitivity of calcium-sensing receptor to Ca^{++} is encouraging in long-term treatment of secondary HPT.

Kidney transplantation can restore metabolic homeostasis in patients with end-stage kidney disease, but more than 25% of patients have persistent elevated PTH one year after transplantation. This condition is known as autonomous HPT (or tertiary HPT). Indications to PTx in tertiary HPT has become more liberal fearing long-term complications. Accurate preoperative imaging studies are always requested, whereas there is no general agreement on the extent of surgery. Surgery is suggested to prevent bone and cardiovascular complications in these patients, and subtotal PTx *versus* total PTx plus autotransplantation are the two available options under discussion [57].

SURGICAL TREATMENT OF ASYMPTOMATIC HYPERPARATHYROIDISM

It has been assessed that all patients with symptomatic primary HPT should undergo surgical treatment, while for symptomatic or minimally symptomatic patients the role of surgery is still debated. The incidence of asymptomatic HPT has changed over the years (Table **2**).

Table 2: Changes of main clinical features in patients with primary hyperparathyroidism. Modified from [14].

Years	Nephrolithiasis	Radiologically evident skeletal disease	Asymptomatic
1930-1970	51-57%	10-23%	0.6-18%
1970-2000	17-37%	1.4-14%	22-80%

The introduction of multichannel biochemical analyzers in early 70s, allowed routine estimation of calcium levels and identification of several cases of asymptomatic PHPT [14]. Before 1970s clinical presentation was mainly based on nephrolithiasis, while in the last decades the clinical features have shifted to a less symptomatic or even asymptomatic HPT, which currently accounts for about 85% of patients. Furthermore, differences between Countries has been reported, since the clinical appearance of primary HPT in Europe is typically more "symptomatic" than in the USA [58].

A recent Consensus Conference updated previous indications for when surgery is recommended, and new guidelines (Table **11**) have been suggested [59, 60]. Serum calcium concentration, urinary calcium excretion, and bone density can show evidence for progression of the disease in at least one fourth of patients with asymptomatic primary HPT, but new pharmacologic approaches, such as bisphosphonates and calcimimetics, are also available [61] (see Chapter 8). In patients who do not undergo surgery, serum calcium and creatinine should be tested annually, and bone density (at 3 sites) every 1 or 2 years [60].

In any case, after curative surgery serum calcium, PTH and 24 h urinary calcium return to normal, indicators of bone resorption normalize, and bone mineral density increases significantly [62, 63]. Renal disease shows a variable response to surgery, while no significant improvement in cardiovascular disease has been reported. One of the most important questions concerns whether PTx decreases the risk of future fracture. Recently, some cohort studies found that a risk of fracture declines after PTx, and the effect is independent of age and initial serum calcium and PTH levels [14, 60]. Neurological and neuropsychiatric symptoms are difficult to diagnose and quantify. However, in a recent study, all eight domains of the SF-36 (version 2) score significantly improved, for up to one year, irrespective of whether the patients met the NIH operative criteria, confirming that these symptoms are disabling for the patients [14, 64].

CONCLUSIONS

Primary HPT is the main cause of hypercalcemia, and suitable for surgical treatment in most cases. Considering the significant improvements of clinical features of the disease after successful PTx, and the effectiveness and safety of minimally invasive surgical techniques, surgery should be suggested both in symptomatic patients and in those with asymptomatic or minimally symptomatic primary HPT. However, each patient should be referred to an experienced parathyroid surgeon or endocrinologist, with the aim of having a better definition of the disease, and suggestion for treatment.

REFERENCES

[1]   DeLellis RA, Xia L. Paraneoplastic endocrine syndromes: a review. Endocr Pathol 2003; 14: 303-317.
[2]   Clines GA, Guise TA. Hypercalcemia of malignancy and basic research on mechanism responsible for osteolytic and osteoblastic metastasis to bone. Endocr Relat Cancer 2005; 12: 549-583.
[3]   Lumachi F, Brunello A, Roma A, Basso U. Cancer-induced hypercalcemia. Anticancer Res 2009; 29: 1551-1556.
[4]   Grill V, Martin TJ. Hypercalcemia of malignancy. Rev Endocr Metabol Dis 2000; 1: 253-263.
[5]   Carney JA. The glandulae parathyroideae of Ivar Sandström. Contributions from two continents. Am J Surg Pathol 1996; 20: 1123-1144.
[6]   Askanazy M. Ueber Ostitis Deformans ohne Osteoides gewebe. Arb Path Anat Inst Tübingen (Leipzig) 1904; 4: 398-422.

[7]   Giddings CE, Rimmer J, Weir N. History of parathyroid gland surgery: an historical case series. J Laryngol Otol 2009; 123: 1075-1081.

[8]   Åkerström G, Malmaeus J, Bergström R. Surgical anatomy of human parathyroid glands. Surgery 1984; 95: 14-21.

[9]   Varga I, Pospisilova V, Gmitterova K, Galfiova P, Polak S, Galbavy S. The phylogenesis and the ontogenesis of the human pharyngeal region focused on the thymus, parathyroid, and thyroid glands. Neuro Endocrinol Lett 2008; 29: 837-845.

[10]   Lumachi F, Marzola MC, Zucchetta P, Cecchin D, Bui F. Different operative protocols for minimally invasive radioguided parathyroidectomy. A randomized prospective study. Ann Surg Oncol 2004; 11: S103-S104.

[11]   Åkerström G, Grimelius R, Johansson H, Lindquist H, Pertoft H, Bergström R. The parenchymal cell mass in normal human parathyroid glands. Acta Pathol Microbiol Scand 1981; 89: 367-75.

[12]   Verdonk CA, Edis AJ. Parathyroid "double adenomas": fact or fiction? Surgery 1981; 90: 523-526.

[13]   Shindo ML, WU JC, Park EE. Surgical anatomy of the recurrent laryngeal nerve revisited. Otolaryngol Head Neck Surg 2005; 133: 514-519.

[14]   Fraser WD. Hyperparathyroidism. Lancet 2009; 374: 145-158.

[15]   Iglesias P, Díez JJ. Current treatments in the management of patients with primary hyperparathyroidism. Postgrad Med J 2009; 85: 15-23.

[16]   Harman CR, Grant CS, Hay ID, *et al*. Indications, technique, and efficacy of alcohol injection of enlarged parathyroid glands in patients with primary hyperparathyroidism. Surgery 1998; 124: 1011-1019.

[17]   Vergès B, Cercueil JP, Jacob D, Vaillant G, Brun JM. Traitement des adénomes parathyroïdiens par alcoolisation sous contrôle échographique. Ann Chir 2000; 125: 457-460.

[18]   Miller DL, Doppman JL, Chang R, *et al*. Angiographic ablation of parathyroid adenomas: lessons from a 10-year experience. Radiology 1987; 165: 601-607.

[19]   Cook GJR, Fogelman I, Reidy JF. Succesfull repeat transcatheter ablation of a mediastinal parathyroid adenoma 6 years after alcohol embolization. Cardiovasc Intervent Radiol 1997; 20: 314-316.

[20]   Low RA, Katz AD. Parathyroidectomy via bilateral cervical exploration: a retrospective review of 866 cases. Head Neck 1998; 20: 583-587.

[21]   Nottingham JM, Brown JJ, Bynoe RP, Bell RM, Haynes JL. Bilateral neck exploration for primary hyperparathyroidism. Am Surg 1993; 59: 115-119.

[22]   Russel CF, Edis AJ. Surgery for primary hyperparathyroidism: experience with 500 consecutive cases and evaluation of the role of surgery in the asymptomatic patient. Br J Surg 1982; 69: 244-247.

[23]   Wang C-A. Surgical management of primary hyperparathyroidism. Curr Probl Surg 1985; 22: 1-50.

[24]   Tibblin S, Bondeson A-G, Ljungberg O. Unilateral parathyroidectomy in hyperpara-thyroidism due to single adenoma. Ann Surg 1982; 195: 245-252.

[25]   Pellizzo MR, Pagetta C, Piotto A, *et al*. Surgical treatment of primary hyperparathyroidism: from bilateral neck exploration to minimally invasive surgery. Minerva Endocrinol 2008; 33: 85-93.

[26]   Sackett WR, Barraclough B, Reeve TS, Delbridge LW. Worldwide trends in the surgical treatment of primary hyperparathyroidism in the era of minimally invasive parathyroidectomy. Arch Surg 2002; 137: 1055-1059.

[27]   Gagner M. Endoscopic subtotal parathyroidectomy in patients with primary hyperpara-thyroidism. Br J Surg 1996; 83: 875.

[28]   Inabnet WB, Fulla Y, Richard B, Bonnichou P, Icard P, Chapuis Y. Unilateral neck exploration under local anesthesia: the approach of choice for asymptomatic primary hyperparathyroidism. Surgery 1999; 126: 1004-1010.

[29]   Kaplan EL, Yashiro T, Salti G. Primary hyperparathyroidism in the 1990s. Choice of surgical procedures for the disease. Ann Surg 1992; 215: 300-317.

[30]   Sebag F, Hubbard JG, Maweja S, Misso C, Tardivet L, Henry JF. Negative preoperative localization studies are highly predictive of multiglandular disease in sporadic primary hyperparathyroidism. Surgery 2003; 134: 1038-1041.

[31]   Stawicki SP, El Chaar M, Baillie DR, Jaik NP, Estrada FP. Correlation between biochemical testing, pathology findngs and preoperative sestamibi scans: a retrospective study of the minimally invasive radioguided parathyroidectomy (MIRP) approach. Nucl Med Rev Cent East Eur 2007; 10: 82-86.

[32]   Lumachi F, Zucchetta P, Marzola MC, *et al*. Advantages of combined technetium-99m-sestamibi scintigraphy and high-resolution ultrasonography in parathyroid localization: comparative study in 91 patients with primary hyperparathyroidism. Eur J Endocrinol 2000; 143: 755-760.

[33]   Lumachi F, Ermani M, Basso SMM, *et al*. Localization of parathyroid tumours in the minimally invasive era: which technique should be chosen ? Population-based analysis of 253 patients undergoing parathyroidectomy and factors affecting parathyroid gland detection. Endocr Relat Cancer 2001; 8: 63-69.

[34]   Haber RS, Kim CK, Inabnet WB. Ultrasonography for preoperative localization of enlarged parathyroid glands in primary hyperparathyroidism: comparison with 99-m-technetium sestamibi scintigraphy. Clin Endocrinol 2002; 57: 241-249.

[35]   Reeve TS, Babidge WJ, Parkyn RF, *et al*. Minimally invasive surgery for primary hyperparathyroidism. Systematic review. Arch Surg 2000; 135: 481-487.

[36]   Aarum S, Nordenström J, Reihnér E, *et al*. Operation for primary hyperparathyroidism: the new versus the old order. Scand J Surg 2007; 96: 26-30.

[37]   Mitchell J, Milas M, Barbosa G, Sutton J, Berber E, Siperstein A. Avoidable reoperations for thyroid and parathyroid surgery: effect of hospital volume. Surgery 2008; 144: 899-906.

[38]   Reidel MA, Schilling T, Graf S, *et al*. Localization of hyperfunctioning parathyroid glands by selective venous sampling in reoperation for primary or secondary hyperparathyroidism. Surgery 2006; 140: 907-913.

[39]   Harrison BJ. What steps should be considered in the patient that had a negative cervical exploration for primary hyperparathyroidism? Clin Endocrinol 2009; 71: 624-627.

[40]   Miccoli P, Berti P, Materazzi G, Massi M, Picone A, Minuto MN. Results of video-assisted parathyroidectomy: single institution's six-year experience. World J Surg 2004; 28: 1216-1218.

[41]   Henry JF, Sebag F, Tamagnini P, Forman C, Silaghi H. Endoscopic parathyroid surgery: results of 356 consecutive procedures. World J Surg 2004; 28: 1219-1223.

[42]   Lee KE, Kim HY, Park WS, *et al*. Postauricolar and axillary approach endoscopic neck surgery: a new technique. World J Surg 2009; 33: 767-772.

[43]   Mihai R, Barczynski M, Iacobone M, Sitges-Serra A. Surgical strategy for sporadic primary hyperparathyroidism an evidence-based approach to surgical strategy, patient selection, surgical access, and reoperations. Langenbecks Arch Surg 2009; 394: 785-798.

[44]   Palazzo FF, Delbridge LW. Minimal-access/minimally invasive parathyroidectomy for primary hyperparathyroidism. Surg Clin N Am 2004; 84: 717-734.

[45]   Sosa JA, Powe NR, Levine MA, Udelsman R, Zeiger MA. Profile of a clinical practice: thresholds for surgery and surgical outcomes for patients with primary hyperparathyroidism: a national survey of endocrine surgeons. J Clin Endocrinol Metab 1998; 83: 2658-2665.

[46]   Harrison BJ, Triponez F. Intraoperative adjuncts in surgery for primary hyperparathyroidism. Langenbecks Arch Surg 2009; 394: 799-809.

[47]   Bergenfelz AOJ, Jansson SKG, Wallin GK, *et al*. Impact of modern techniques on short-term outcome after surgery for primary hyperparathyroidism: a multicenter study comprising 2,708 patients. Langenbecks Arch Surg 2009; 394: 851-860.

[48]   Chan RK, Ibrahim SI, Pil P, Tanasijevic M, Moore FD. Validation of a method to replace frozen section during parathyroid exploration by using the rapid parathyroid hormone assay on parathyroid aspirates. Arch Surg 2005; 140: 371-373.

[49]   Lumachi F, Ermani M, Marino F, *et al*: Relationship of AgNOR counts and nuclear DNA content to survival in patients with parathyroid carcinoma. Endocr Relat Cancer 2004; 11: 563-569.

[50]   Lumachi F, Ermani M, Marino F, *et al*. PCNA-Li, Ki 67 immunostaining, p53 activity and histopathological variables in predicting the clinical outcome in patients with parathyroid carcinoma. Anticancer Res 2006; 26: 1305-1308.

[51]   Shoback D, Marcus R, Bikle D, Strewler G. Mineral metabolism & metabolic bone disease. In: Greenspan FS & Gardner DG, Eds. Basic & Clinical Endocrinology. New York, Lange Medical Books/McGraw Hill, 2001; pp. 237-333.

[52]   Busaidy NL, Jimenez C, Habra MA, *et al*. Parathyroid carcinoma: a 22-year experience. Head Neck 2004; 26: 716-726.

[53]   Okamoto T, Iihara M, Obara T, Tsukada T. Parathyroid carcinoma: etiology, diagnosis, and treatment. World J Surg 2009; 33: 2343-2354.

[54] Lumachi F, Basso SMM, Basso U. Parathyroid cancer: etiology, clinical presentation and treatment. Anticancer Res 2006; 26: 4803-4808.

[55] Munson ND, Foote RL, Northcutt RC, *et al.* Parathyroid carcinoma: is there a role for adjuvant radiation therapy? Cancer 2003; 98: 2378-2384.

[56] Iacobone M, Ruffolo C, Lumachi F, Favia G. Results of iterative surgery for persistent and recurrent parathyroid carcinoma. Langenbecks Arch Surg 2005; 390: 385-390.

[57] Triponez F, Clark OH, Vanrenthergem Y, Evenepoel P. Surgical treatment of persistent hyperparathyroidism after renal transplantation. Ann Surg 2008; 248: 18-30.

[58] Khan AA, Bilezikian JP, Potts JT Jr. The diagnosis and management of asymptomatic primary hyperparathyroidism revisited. J Clin Endocrinol Metab 2009; 94: 333-334.

[59] Udelsman R, Pasieka JL, Sturgeon C, Young JEM, Clark OH. Surgery for asymptomatic primary hyperparathyroidism: proceedings of the Third International Workshop. J Clin Endocrinol Metab 2009; 94: 366-372.

[60] Bilezikian JP, Khan AA, Potts JT. Guidelines for the management of asymptomatic primary hyperparathyroidism: summary statement from the Third International Workshop. J Clin Endocrinol Metab 2009; 94: 335-339.

[61] Bilezikian JP, Potts JT jr. Asymptomatic primary hyperparathyroidism: new issues and new questions-bridging the past with the future. J Bone Miner Res 2002; 17(S2): N57-N67.

[62] Lumachi F, Ermani M, Basso SM, *et al.* Short- and long-term changes in bone mineral density of the lumbar spine after parathyroidectomy in patients with primary hyperparathyroidism. Calcif Tissue Int 2003; 73: 44-48.

[63] Lumachi F, Camozzi V, Ermani M, De Lotto F, Luisetto G. Bone mineral density improvement after successful parathyroidectomy in pre-and postmenopausal women with primary hyperparathyroidism. A prospective study. Ann N Y Acad Sci 2008; 1117: 357-261.

[64] Caillard C, Sebag F, Mathonnet M, *et al.* Prospective evaluation of quality of life (SF-36v2) and nonspecific symptoms before and after cure of primary hyperparathyroidism (1-year follow-up). Surgery 2007; 141: 153-159.

CHAPTER 8

Medical Treatment of Hypercalcemia

Valentina Camozzi, Chiara Franzin and Giovanni Luisetto

Department of Medical and Surgical Sciences, University of Padua, 35128 Padova, Italy

Abstract: Hypercalcemia is a relatively common disorder. Primary hyperparathyroidism and malignancy-associated hypercalcemia (MAH) are responsible for more than 90% of all causes of hypercalcemia. General measures of treatment include rehydration and loop diuretics, when renal insufficiency or heart failure is associated. Calcitonin is indicated for the short-term control of severe hypercalcemia, while bisphosphonates are required in the long-term management. The antireabsorptive action of bisphosphonates has been considered the most effective in the disorders characterized by an excessive bone resorption. Both clodronate and pamidronate have been widely used in the past. Recently controlled clinical trials demonstrated the superiority of zoledronate compared with previous treatments. The use of calcimimetic agents has been recently introduced to control hypercalcemia in selected cases of primary hyperparathyroidism. They are used when patients do not meet surgical criteria or surgery is not possible or accepted. Recent studies on cancer-induced bone disease have highlighted the role of receptor activator of nuclear factor-κ ligand (RANKL) as a critical effector of skeletal complications of malignancy. RANKL inhibitors may reduce bone resorption in patients with bone metastases and multiple myeloma. Malignancy-associated hypercalcemia is broadly divided into two categories: humoral MAH and osteolytic MAH. The former refers to the paraneoplastic release of humoral factors, mainly parathyroid hormone-related peptide (PTHrP). A humanized monoclonal antibody against human PTHrP has been generated. It is able to neutralize the PTHrP effects, reducing hypercalcemia in human tumor xenograft animal models.

INTRODUCTION

Hypercalcemia is relatively a common disorder (see Chapter 1), which requires specific treatment in order to control symptoms and prevent the development of organ damage. The symptoms of hypercalcemia are wide-ranging but non specific (see Chapter 2). The most common comparison of hypercalcemia picked up on routine biochemical samples. Serum calcium concentration can be divided into three components: ionized serum calcium (45%), serum calcium complexed to anions (phosphate, sulfate, carbonate, 10%), calcium bound to albumin (45%). Hypercalcemia is defined as a serum calcium >2 standard deviations above the normal mean in a given laboratory, commonly 2.65 mmol/L (10.6 mg/dL) for total serum calcium, and 1.25 mmol/L for ionized serum calcium (see Chapter 5). Hypercalcemic symptoms tend to increase in proportion to the degree of serum concentration, which is regulated by the flux of ionized serum calcium to and from three physiologic compartments: the bone, the intestine, and the kidney (see Chapter 1). Understanding the underlying imbalance of the mechanism is a critical point to define the origin of hypercalcemia, in order to establish the correct

therapeutic strategy. The restriction of dietary calcium intake, but not the use of antiresorptive agents, can be helpful to restore the normal calcium values in case of milk-alkali syndrome or vitamin D intoxication. The problem rises when hypercalcemia is associated with conditions more difficult to treat.

Since, primary hyperparathyroidism (HPT) and malignancy are responsible for more than 90% of all cases of hypercalcemia, greater interest was given in terms of developing the best "strategy" to manage these two critical situations. Currently, the development of a moiety that activates the calcium-sensing receptor (CaSR) mimicking calcium effect on parathyroid (PT) glands, has changed the history of primary HPT. Whereas, the management of cancer-induced hypercalcemia is more complicated.

Malignancy-associated hypercalcemia (MAH) is broadly divided into two categories: humoral MAH, and osteolytic MAH (see Chapter 3). The former refers to the paraneoplastic release of humoral factors, mainly parathyroid hormone-related protein (PTHrP), whereas local osteolytic hypercalcemia refers to the local destruction of bone by tumor with calcium release. There might be considerable overlap between these two mechanisms in the pathogenesis of MAH.

Due to their antiresorptive action, bisphosphonates (BPs) are currently the treatment of choice in cancer related bone disease. However, the clinical efficacy of BPs in MAH is usually short-lived and sometimes incomplete. This is due to the increased distal tubular calcium reabsorption driven by PTHrP.

BISPHOSPHONATES

It is now generally accepted that osteoclast activation plays a key role in the establishment and growth of all bone metastases. Biochemical data indicate that bone resorption is important not only in the lytic, but also in sclerotic lesions. Inhibition of bone resorption is a crucial point to stop the progression of the bone metastatic disease and its complications, such as hypercalcemia.

Mechanism of Action, Affinity and Potency

Bisphosphonates are the major class of drugs for the treatment of bone diseases in bone disorders, characterized by an excessive bone resorption, including cancer related bone disease. Their biological effects were initially correlated to their ability to bind mineral bone surface and inhibit the dissolution of hydroxyapatite (HAP) crystals, as had already been shown for pyrophosphate. Bisphosphonates also act directly on osteoclasts and interfere with specific intracellular biochemical process, such as isoprenoid biosynthesis and subsequent protein prenylation to inhibit cellular activity [1].

The first synthesis of BPs occurred in the 19th century. They are stable analogs of naturally occurring inorganic pyrophosphate, in which a carbon atom replaces the oxygen atom connecting the two phosphates. The resistance to enzymatic or acid hydrolysis is conferred by the carbon atom, which binds two phosphonate groups. These groups are required both for binding bone mineral and for cell-mediated antiresorptive activity. The two side-chains attached to the carbon atom are able to modify the affinity to bone surface and the biochemical potency (R_1 and R_2, respectively) [1].

The binding affinity to HAP is characterized by the attachment to the mineral surface and the duration of the bonding. It is conditioned by the P-C-P structure and by the R_1 side-chain, being greater when R_1 is a hydroxyl (OH) rather than a chlorine substituent, as in clodronate [2]. Due to these features significant differences were observed among BPs. A nitrogen moiety and its position in the alkyl group or heterocyclic ring in R_2 chain can increase the binding ability (Fig. **1**).

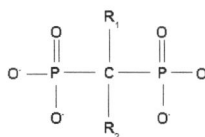

Figure 1: Bisphosphonates basic structure: R_1 and R_2 are the two side-chains attached to the carbon atom are able to modify the affinity to bone surface and the biochemical potency.

The established binding affinity to HAP was in ascending order: clodronate, etidronate, risedronate, ibandronate, alendronate, pamidronate, and zoledronate [1].

Bisphosphonates inhibit bone resorption through intracellular effects on osteoclasts: they impair osteoclast function, and reduce osteoclast resorption. During bone resorption the acidification produced by vacuolar-type proton pump of the osteoclast ruffer border in the microenvironment. Thus, this determines the dissolution of HAP, thereby favoring the detachment of BPs from HAP. The breakdown of extracellular bone matrix is due to the action of proteolytic enzyme. After these changes BPs are taken into osteoclasts by an endocytic mechanism.

Due to their mechanism of action BPs have been subdivided into two major groups: (1) the non-nitrogen containing BPs (nN-BPs), such as clodronate and etidronate, and (2) the nitrogen-containing BPs (N-BPs), such as alendronate and pamidronate (containing an amino group [NH_2]in an alkyl chain), risedronate and zoledronate (containing a nitrogen [N] atom within a heterocyclic ring), and ibandronate, that contains a tertiary nitrogen [2] (Fig. **2**).

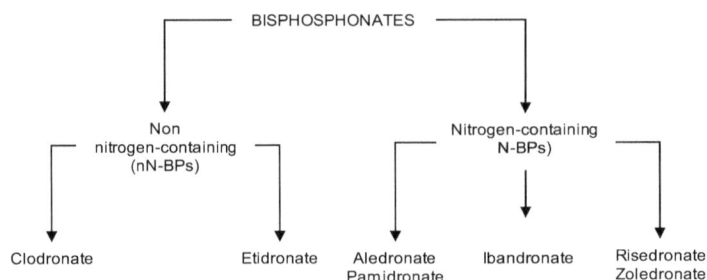

Figure 2: Groups of bisphosphonates.

The nN-BPs are incorporated into non-hydrolyzable β, γ-methylene analogs of adenosine triphosphate (ATP). The intracellular accumulation of these nonhydrolyzable ATP analogs inhibits osteoclast function leading to cell apoptosis. BPs of the second group (N-BPs) interfere in the mevalonate pathway, the same as with cholesterol and other steroids biosynthesis. N-BPs act mainly by interfering with farnesyl pyrophosphate synthase (FPPS). The inhibition of FPPS stops the synthesis of farnesyl pyrophosphate (FPP), which in turn reduces the substrate concentrations of FPP necessary for geranylgeranylpyrophosphate (GGPP) synthase to produce GGPP.

Both FPP and GGPP are required for the lipid modification (prenylation) of small GTPases that are fundamental signaling proteins for the function and survival of osteoclasts. Some N-BPs are also characterized by containing a heterocyclic ring (risedronate, zoledronate) [2]. The heterocyclic N-BPs also inhibit the FPPS enzyme and in addition stabilizes conformational changes that magnify their inhibitory potency (Fig. **3**).

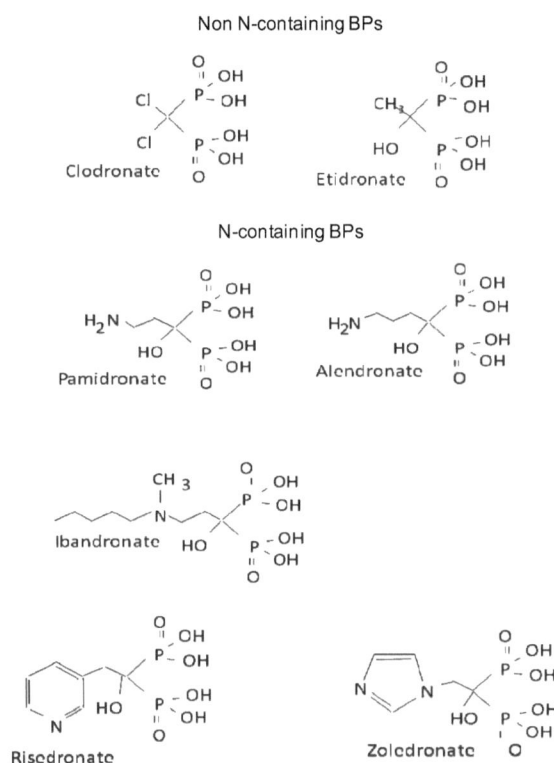

Figure 3: The figure shows the formula of the more commonly used bisphosphonates. Non- nitrogen containing bisphosphonates (nN-BPs): clodronate and etidronate. Nitrogen containing bisphosphonates (N-BPs) alendronate

and pamidronate, that contain an amino group (NH) in an alkyl chain; risedronate and zoledronate, that contains a nitrogen (N) atom within a heterocyclic ring, and ibandronate that contains a tertiary nitrogen.

The ascending order of FPPS enzyme inhibition is: etidronate, clodronate, pamidronate, alendronate, ibandronate, risedronate, and zoledronate [1]. The different binding to the bone, as well as the inhibitory potency for FPPS, can affect BPs action in terms of greater suppression and longer persistence of the effects. It is difficult to establish the half-life of these compounds, due to the persistence of the drug within the mineral phase. The release of BPs from bone correlates with bone turnover and is dependent on chemical detachment from HAP surface and osteoclastic resorption.

The binding of BPs to HAP surface is a reversible process that is conditioned by the extracellular fluid levels. When the extracellular fluid levels are high, the uptake of BPs by the bone will occur, while the detachment will be determined with low levels. The diffusion through a deep site will be slower. The BPs affinity for HAP can affect the diffusion of the drug into the bone.

The BPs with the highest affinity for HAP have a higher adsorption, lower desorption and lower ability to diffuse through other skeletal sites. The release of BPs during the osteoclastic resorption contributes to the recirculation of the drugs after cessation of administration. BPs recycling would extend the effects of the treatment, although the accelerated resorption promotes the BPs' disappearance from bone.

Clinical Use of Bisphosphonates

Bisphosphonates are used to treat different diseases, all characterized by increased bone resorption: (1) osteoporosis, (2) Paget's disease of bone, also called *osteitis deformans*, in which predominating bone resorption is usually accompanied by an adequate increase in bone formation. This is accompanied by replacement of normal marrow by fibrous connective tissue, and (3) cancer-related bone impairment, especially observed in patients with MAH. The development of the clinical use of BPs led to different choice of the treatment and management of a specific medical situation.

Thirty years ago, BPs were started to be used as therapeutic agents in oncology for the treatment of skeletal-related bone complications, such as accelerated bone resorption and hypercalcemia. Currently, BPs are the drugs of choice in cancer-related bone disease since they are employed in the treatment of multiple myeloma and metastases from breast cancer, prostate cancer, lung cancer, renal cell carcinoma, and other solid tumors [1-3]. The clinical pharmacology of BPs is characterized by low intestinal absorption (less than 1%), so that the parenteral administration is preferable to reach a defined action rapidly.

Following the intravenous administration of a BP, about 25-40% of the injected dose is excreted by the kidney, and the remainder is taken up by bone.

The decrease of serum calcium occurs after 24-48 hours, and the normalization of its levels is obtained within 7 days. In life-threatening hypercalcemia, rehydration and high doses of parenteral calcitonin, should be concomitantly administered together with the BPs during the first 24 hours. Zoledronate and pamidronate are currently approved in the USA, while in Europe clodronate and ibandronate are also approved [4].

The recommended doses are: clodronate 300 mg, pamidronate 90 mg, ibandronate 6 mg, zoledronate 4 mg, as a single infusion every 3-4 weeks, except clodronate that must be infused daily for 5 consecutive days. The intravenous BPs administration covers a period ranging from 15 minutes (zoledronate) to 2-4 hours (clodronate, pamidronate), depending on the moiety. Intravenous ibandronate can be administered by bolus injection over a few minutes, without increasing the risk of nephrotoxicity. All the molecules achieve normocalcemia in 80-90% of cases [5]. The clinical efficacy of BPs in MAH sometimes may be incomplete, due to the increased distal tubular calcium reabsorption driven by PTHrP [6].

The superiority of pamidronate over clodronate in patients with MAH has been demonstrated in a randomized trial. Both clodronate and pamidronate reduced serum calcium levels at the same rate, but the median duration of action of clodronate was 2 weeks compared with 4 weeks for pamidronate [7].

Recently, controlled clinical trials have shown the superiority of i.v. zoledronate compared with previous BP treatments in the management of the skeletal complications secondary to multiple myeloma, or a broad range of solid tumors, including breast, prostate and lung carcinomas [8]. Metastatic bone lesions can result in substantial morbidity, including severe bone pain and complications, such as pathological fractures, spinal cord compression, and potentially life-threatening hypercalcemia. As a consequence, patients frequently require surgical intervention or radiotherapy.

Without BPs' therapy, patients with osteolytic lesions from advanced breast cancer may suffer skeletal complications at an average rate of 3-4 events per year. During a 2-year study period in the placebo arm of an earlier pamidronate trial, 52% of patients, with predominantly osteolytic bone lesions secondary to breast carcinoma, developed pathologic fractures, and 13% experienced hypercalcemia [9, 10]. In a long-term (25 months) study comparing efficacy and safety of zoledronic acid (4 mg) and pamidronate disodium (90 mg) in patients with advanced multiple myeloma or breast carcinoma, zoledronate reduced the overall risk of developing skeletal complications, including hypercalcemia by an additional 16% (p=0.030), with no increase in the risk of renal impairment [9]. Intravenous ibandronate can also be used in these situations. Whether or not, intravenous ibandronate will be a therapeutic advance over intravenous zoledronate or pamidronate is still an open question. Head-to-head randomized controlled trials are necessary to clear this speculation [11].

Across different solid tumors, the prevalence of bone metastases is highest in breast and prostate cancer (65% and 75%, respectively), followed by thyroid (60%), lung (40%), and bladder cancer (30-40%). To date, intravenous N-BPs are the treatment of choice for reducing, delaying and preventing skeletal complications associated with cancer bone involvement [12].

Adverse Effects and Safety

Gastrointestinal problems, local reaction at the injection site, and uveitis are minor complications. Flu-like symptoms may occur during the first administration of BPs, due to the induction of an acute phase reaction. Acetaminophen or paracetamol can control these effects, that are commonly transient. Short-term asymptomatic or minimally symptomatic hypocalcemia and hypophosphatemia may also occur. Due to their kidney excretion, these drugs should be carefully administered in patient with renal insufficiency. In subjects with mild to moderate renal impairment, [creatinine clearance (CrCl) 30-60 ml/min] lower doses and longer infusion time are recommended. In patients with evidence of renal function impairment during treatment, the N-BPs administration should be withdrawn, and only resumed when serum creatinine returns within 10% of baseline [12].

Osteonecrosis of the jaw (ONJ) is a disease characterized by exposed bone in the maxillofacial region, that does not heal. Additional signs and symptoms include pain, swelling, paresthesia, soft tissue ulceration and suppuration. It is an uncommon but potentially serious complication, predominantly seen in patients receiving high doses of potent i.v. N-BPs, mostly observed during treatment for multiple myeloma or breast cancer [13]. A retrospective analysis of about 4,000 patients with multiple myeloma and breast cancer treated with intravenous BPs was conducted between 1996 and 2004. ONJ developed in 1.2% of patients with breast cancer, and 2.4% in those with myeloma. Other studies showed a larger percentage of ONJ in cancer patients (about 9%), and the real incidence of this occurrence is yet to be established [14].

The etiology of ONJ is still unclear but likely multifactorial. Actinomyces has been found frequently in these lesions, indicating that osteomyelitis at sites of dental/jaw trauma may contribute to such complications. ONJ seems to be time and dose-dependent on BPs treatment, and there is a strong association with dental surgery. Other potential risk factors include chemotherapy, glucocorticoids, and lack of oral hygiene. Before starting i.v. N-BPs administration, patients should have a dental examination and any treatment required. Antibiotic prophylaxis, before and after dental intervention, can limit the occurrence of this complication.

NON BISPHOSPHONATES DRUGS

These paragraphs will point out the general measures that must be taken in the management of hypercalcemia, and the therapeutic options before the "bisphosphonate era".

Hydration and Diuretics

Dehydration is a frequent complication of hypercalcemia. Restoration volume repletion should be the first measure to be taken during the treatment of hypercalcemia of any cause. An excess of calcium causes a potent diuretic effect that is associated to loss of sodium. The kidney increases its tubular reabsorption of both sodium and calcium, that in turn worsens hypercalcemia (see Chapter 1). The continuous infusion (3-6 liters over 24-48 hours) of saline (NaCl 0.9%) can lower serum calcium concentration by approximately 1.0-3.0 mg/dL (0.25 mmol/L-0.75 mmol/L) by decreasing the concomitant reabsorption of sodium and calcium, and promoting the sodium-linked calcium diuresis in the proximal renal tubule [4, 15].

Loop diuretics, particularly furosemide, are traditionally used because they increase urinary calcium excretion. Begining in 1970, reports of the use of furosemide to increase calciuresis are reported, and doses ranging from 10 to 80 mg/h are commonly recommended [16]. Recently, their effective utility to control hypercalcemia is under discussion since scientific evidence to support their use is lacking. Because of their concomitant natriuretic effects, loop diuretics must carefully be administered. This therapeutic approach requires close monitoring of serum-urinary electrolytes and blood pressure. This should be restricted to patients at risk of volume overload, such as elderly patients with compromised cardiac and/or renal function.

Calcitonin

Calcitonin is a 32-aminoacid peptide originating from the thyroid C parafollicular cells. Osteoclasts are the major targets for its action. This peptide directly and rapidly causes a loss of the ruffled border of osteoclasts, inducing contraction and inhibition of osteoclast motility. It reduces the number of osteoclasts, and interferes with their differentiation from precursor cells and fusion of mononucleated precursors to form multinucleated osteoclasts in bone marrow cultures.

Calcitonin also inhibits the acid secretion of osteoclasts, reducing both synthesis and release of tartrate-resistant acid phosphatase (TRAP). Such cellular effects lead to a potent antiresorptive action. It also enhances calcium excretion by the kidney, and inhibits tubular calcium resorption [17, 18]. This peptide is a valuable approach associated with rehydration in the immediate short-term management of severe symptomatic hypercalcemia. It acts rapidly, by decreasing calcium levels within 2 hours after administration. Salmon calcitonin is more potent than both human and porcine ones.

Various regimens have been used, although the dose-response relationship seems to range between 25-50 IU (4-8 IU/kg) every 8-12 hours, by subcutaneous and intravenous injection [15]. Its rapid activity is useful in controlling hypercalcemia during the first 24-48 h after administration. Many patients escape control after 2-3 days due to down-regulation of calcitonin receptors on the osteoclast. In the treatment of MAH, calcitonin should be combined with BPs. They have time to take effect and their action in the control of hypercalcemia begins when the calcitonin effect declines.

Steroids

Glucocorticoids have been used in the past to treat hypercalcemia, especially in patients with hematologic malignancies. At present, their use is restricted to the treatment of hypercalcemia due to ectopic endogenous production of $1,25(OH)_2D_3$, such as sarcoidosis. However, they are rarely effective in hypercalcemia due to solid tumors (lymphoma, disgerminoma).

Prednisone (20-40 mg daily, orally) or hydrocortisone (120 mg daily, orally or intravenously) are commonly administered. Serum levels of $[1,25(OH)_2]D_3$, as well as serum calcium decrease usually within 3 to 5 days [4]. Failure to normalize serum calcium levels after two weeks leads the clinicians to exclude the possibility of a coexisting disorder, including HPT, carcinoma, lymphoma and myeloma. Once calcium levels become normal, glucocorticoids dosage can be reduced over a period of 4 to 6 weeks [19].

NEW DRUGS & FUTURE PERSPECTIVES

Calcimimetics

Calcimimetics are molecules that activate the calcium-sensing receptor (CaSR) by mimicking calcium effect, in particular on PT cells. They decrease serum levels of parathyroid hormone (PTH) and calcium, with a leftward shift in the set point for calcium-regulated PTH secretion. Based on the available clinical data, calcimimetic cinacalcet (Mimpara © Amgen Inc. Zug, Switzerland) is approved for the treatment of secondary HPT in patients with end-stage renal inefficiency/insufficiency on maintenance dialysis therapy, as part of a therapeutic regimen including phosphate binders and/or vitamin D sterols, and for the reduction of hypercalcemia in patients with primary HPT, and PT carcinoma [20].

Parathyroidectomy is the only definitive treatment for primary HPT, and recommended for patients with moderate-to-severe diseases. However, the majority of patients with primary HPT do not meet the surgical criteria, and some subjects refuse an intervention or have contraindications. Recently, new guidelines for the medical management and follow-up of asymptomatic primary HPT have been established (see Chapter 2). Bisphosphonates, hormone replacement therapy, and raloxifene are proposed to protect bone damage due to the PTH excess, while calcimimetics are the only choice to control the derived hypercalcemia [21].

The ability to decrease serum calcium and PTH levels was evaluated in two randomized, double blind, dose finding studies in patients with primary HPT. Serum calcium levels fell by over 50% 2-4 hours after cinacalcet administration in a dose dependent manner, without increasing urinary calcium excretion. In a longer follow-up period, the normalization of serum calcium levels was demonstrated in 73% of treated patient *versus* 5% of the placebo group after 12 months. PTH levels fell by a modest amount (7.6%), but were significantly lower than that of untreated group [22]. Calcimimetic was used also in case of severe hypercalcemia due to PT carcinoma refractory to general management (rehydratation, loop diuretics, BPs, calcitonin). Although calcium serum levels did not normalize after administration, they were lower than the admission, and acutely responsive to change in calcimimetic doses [23].

In patients with end-stage renal insufficiency on maintenance dialysis and secondary HPT, the recommended starting dose for adults is 30 mg once per day. Cinacalcet should be titrated every 2 to 4 weeks, to a maximum dose of 180 mg once daily to achieve a target PTH. In dialyzed patients, the dose should be between 150-300 pg/mL (15.9-31.8 pmol/L) in the intact PTH assay. Serum calcium levels should be monitored frequently, and within one week of initiation or dose adjustment of the drug [24]. Once the maintenance dose has been established, serum calcium should be measured monthly. If serum calcium levels decrease below the normal range, appropriate steps should be taken, including the adjustment of concomitant therapy.

In patients with functioning PT carcinoma, as well as in those with primary HPT, the treatment should not be initiated when the serum calcium (corrected for albumin) is below the lower limit of the normal range. The recommended starting dose of cinacalcet for adults is 30 mg twice a day. The dose of cinacalcet should be titrated every 2 to 4 weeks, through sequential doses of 30 mg twice daily, 60 mg twice daily, 90 mg twice daily, and 90 mg three or four times daily, as necessary to reduce serum calcium concentration to or below the upper limit of normal. The maximum dose used in clinical trials was 90 mg four times daily. Serum calcium should be measured within 1 week after initiation or dose adjustment of cinacalcet. Once, maintenance dose levels have been established, serum calcium should be measured every 2 to 3 months. After titration to the maximum dose of cinacalcet, serum calcium should be periodically monitored. If clinically relevant reductions in serum calcium are not maintained, discontinuation of therapy should be considered. After oral administration of cinacalcet, maximum plasma concentration is achieved in approximately 2 to 6 hours. Based on between-study comparisons, the absolute bioavailability of cinacalcet in fasted subjects has been estimated to be about 20-25%. Administration of this drug with food results in approximately 50-80% increase in bioavailability. Increases in plasma cinacalcet concentration are similar, regardless of the fat content of the meal. Nausea, vomiting, and hypocalcemia are the only associated adverse effects reported [20].

In patients with tertiary HPT, cinacalcet was administered at individual doses in kidney allograft recipients in prospective studies, with normalization of calcium serum levels, and decrease of plasma PTH levels. Most patients were treated with 30 mg daily with persistence of calcium normalization during a follow up period of 6-12 months. Ongoing clinical analysis in this situation will contribute to better defining the long-term efficiency and safety, since surgery is still the treatment of choice in tertiary HPT.

Denosumab

The receptor activator of nuclear factor-κ (RANKL) and the RANKL/RANKL/osteoprotegerin (OPG) system is a critical determinant of bone remodeling. The RANKL ligand, when bound to RANKL receptors on the surface of osteoclasts precursors, promotes osteoclastogenesis. Osteoprotegerin, a soluble decoy receptor for RANKL, inhibits osteoclast formation. RANKL and OPG are both expressed by osteoblasts and bone marrow stromal cells. The RANKL/OPG ratio imbalance plays a fundamental role in bone remodeling impairment.

Recent studies on cancer-induced bone disease pathophysiology have highlighted the role of RANKL as an interesting effector of skeletal complications of malignancy. Based on preclinical research, the RANKL inhibition is able to block osteoclast activity, survival, and differentiation, providing a specific and novel approach to treating cancer-induced bone lesions in humans, whether they are primarily lytic, mixed lytic/blastic, or purely blastic [25, 26]. There are no published data on the direct alteration of RANKL signaling in MAH, but there is a lot of evidence that tumor products, such as PTHrP, that mediate hypercalcemia, stimulate RANKL, and down-regulates its decoy receptor OPG. It has become clear that the tropism of certain tumors to colonize bone is dependent by the bone microenvironment. As osteoclasts resorb bone, a variety of growth factors, such as transforming growth factor-β (TGF-β), fibroblast growth factors (FGFs), platelet-derived growth factors (PDGFs), bone morphogenetic proteins (BMPs), and insulin-like growth factor-1 (IGF-1) are activated and released into bone microenvironment. Elevated TGF-β does not appear to affect tumor growth, but rather leads to the production of PTHrP by cancer cells, thus establishing a continuously destructive cycle, through upregulation of RANKL, accelerating bone resorption. The release of growth factors through bone resorption allows the establishment and progression of the tumor within the skeleton, determining a vicious cycle [26] (Fig. **4**).

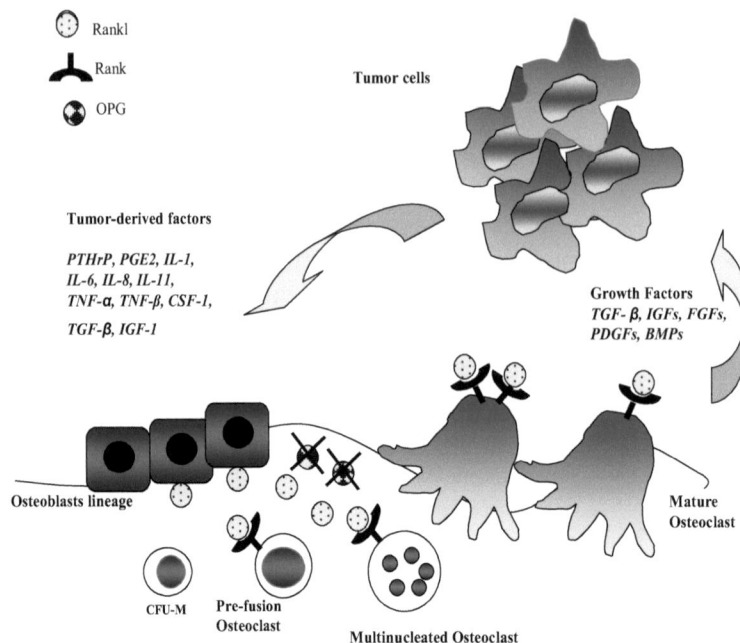

Figure 4: Bone microenvironment and the vicious cycle. The figure illustrates many factors that reciprocally stimulate osteoblast and osteoclast activity and tumor cells growth and survival in the bone microenvironment. Parathyroid hormone-related protein (PTHrP) induces both the production of receptor activator of nuclear factor-κ ligand (RANKL) and down regulation of osteoprotegerin (OPG) production by osteoblasts, thereby stimulating osteoclastogenesis.

Recent experimental data suggest that the RANKL pathway may play a role in bone cancer involvement, also independently from osteoclasts action. Bone-derived RANKL seems to act as a chemoattractant to bone for RANK-expressing cancer cells, inducing invasion and migration of cancer into the bone [27]. Inhibition of RANKL *in vivo* is very effective in reducing bone destruction in murine models of breast cancer, myeloma and prostate cancer. In prostate cancer both osteoblastic and osteolytic lesions respond to the treatment. RANKL inhibition is also effective in animal model of MAH, reducing serum calcium levels significantly more than either zoledronate or pamidronate.

Recently, a fully humanized anti-RANKL antibody, denosumab, has been developed. Denosumab has demonstrated the reduction of bone resorption in patients with solid tumor bone metastases and multiple myeloma in preliminary clinical studies, also reducing some of the tumor-associated *sequelae*, including hypercalcemia [26, 28, 29].

Denosumab exhibited non-linear, dose-dependent pharmacokinetics. Following subcutaneous administration, this drug showed rapid and prolonged absorption, with serum levels that were detectable as early as 1 hour postdose, and average maximum serum concentrations occurring between 7 and 21 days postdose. The suppression of bone turnover was dose dependent, and an administering regimen of 120 mg subcutaneously every 4 weeks was the most effective. This dosage rapidly suppressed the urinary marker of bone resorption N-telopeptide (uNTx), and is now being evaluated in phase III trials.

RANK is expressed on the surface of T-cells and dendritic cells, and inhibition of RANKL theoretically suggests a risk of immune system imbalance. Clinical trials did not show clinically significant immune system adverse events. There are conflicting concerns about potential interference with the inhibition of

RANKL and the pro-apoptotic factor TRIAL. To date, the inhibition does not appear to increase the incidence of neoplasm. The most common adverse events seem to be related to cellulitis and cutaneous rush [30].

Recently, in phase II of the clinical studies, denosumab was compared in patients with bone metastases and multiple myeloma *naïve* to intravenous N-BPs therapy (n=255), and those with elevated levels of the urinary uNTx despite ongoing i.v. N-BPs treatment (n=111). Patients were randomly selected to receive i.v. N-BPs every 4 weeks, subcutaneous denosumab (30, 120, 180 mg), or denosumab every 12 weeks (60 or 180 mg). Zoledronic acid was the most commonly N-BPs used (90%) in both studies. Patients were treated for 25 weeks and underwent 32-week follow-up after treatment. Daily supplementation of calcium (500 mg) and vitamin D (400 IU) were given.

The cutoff value for uNTx < 50 nmol BCE/mmol creatinine was defined on pre-existing data suggesting that uNTx > 50 nmol BCE/mmol creatinine correlated with an increased risk for skeletal related events and cancer progression. Both denosumab and N-BPs caused a rapid reduction of uNTx (-75% and -71%, respectively) in naïve patients. Notably, in patients with high uNTx despite the previous BPs treatment, denosumab reduced the resorption marker after switching therapy, while uNTx remained high in patients that continued BPS (-80%, and 56% respectively). The persistence of high bone resorption markers in patients continuing N-BPs treatment suggest that osteoclasts are still functioning. After switching therapy, the incidence of the related skeletal complication was reduced in the denosumab treated group as compared to the patients continuing BPs [31]. This result highlighted that the distinct mechanism of action causes different effects on bone metabolism. Bisphosphonates act by inhibiting osteoclasts ability to bone resorption, while denosumab acts by inhibiting the binding of RANKL to RANK. This blocks the formation, maturation and survival of osteoclasts that seem completely eradicated from the bone environment.

Taken into account the limited experience, to date, few cases of ONJ have been reported. Anyway, RANKL inhibitors are not stored in bone like BPs, and the suppression of bone turnover is reversible in very little time. RANKL inhibitor seems to be a promising opportunity to manage cancer-related bone complications. Studies with adequate power and duration will define the real efficacy and safety of denosumab.

Parathyroid Hormone-Related Protein Antibody

Parathyroid hormone-related protein was identified as a causative factor of humoral MAH [32]. While PTH activates both bone formation and bone resorption, PTHrP activates mainly osteoclasts, stimulating the production of RANKL by osteoblasts. Thus leading to the destructive vicious cycle above described.

Both PTH and PTHrP bind to the PTH-receptor 1 (PTH1R), a G protein coupled receptor expressing in a wide variety of tissues that stimulates bone resorption and renal reabsorption of calcium. Fragments of PTHrP and PTH containing the N-terminal 34 amino acids are fully capable of binding and activating PTH1R. The inhibition of both PTH and PTHrP might determine hypocalcemic effects, while selective inhibition of PTHrP function can normalize hypercalcemia in MAH patients. It was demonstrated that both polyclonal and monoclonal antibodies that neutralized PTHrP had anti-hypercalcemic effects in animal models.

In an attempt to develop a non immunogenic therapeutic agent for the treatment of MAH, a humanized monoclonal antibody against human PTHrP was generated from the mouse monoclonal antibody raised against the human PTHrP (1-34). This amino acid sequence was conserved both in mouse's and rat's PTHrP. The humanized anti-PTHrP antibody was fully capable of neutralizing PTHrP, and to reduce hypercalcemia in human tumor xenograft animal models [33, 34]. Human studies are necessary to confirm these promising preliminary results.

CONCLUSIONS

Although, hypercalcemia is a relatively common disorder, it might become a severe complication in some conditions such as untreated primary HPT and cancer-related skeletal events. Actually, calcimimetics have changed the history of primary HPT when surgery is not possible, although there are no data regarding their long term usage.

The optimal treatment of MAH is still an open question. Bisphosphonates are the drug of choice, at present. The development of potent moieties, in inhibiting osteoclasts action and their persistence in the bone, has allowed the reduction of bone resorption and related complications, with satisfactory, but not conclusive results. Bisphosphonates are still limited to control the MAH effects, that are sustained by PTHrP actions on the bone and the kidney. The inhibitor of RANKL, denosumab, seems to be a promising option, since it may block both the maturation and the survival of osteoclasts. The future utilization of an antibody against PTHrP might close the spectrum.

More recently it has been shown that wingless-type (Wnts) family, a family of glycoproteins that mediate bone development, and Wnt inhibitory Dickkopfs (DKK1) also play a role in malignant bone disease. These promising recent studies might open up to new possibilities of treatment [35,36].

REFERENCES

[1]   Russell RG, Xia Z, Dunford JE, *et al*. Bisphosphonates: an update on mechanisms of action and how these relate to clinical efficacy. Ann N Y Acad Sci 2007 Nov;1117: 209-257.
[2]   Russell RG. Bisphosphonates: from bench to bedside. Ann NY Acad Sci 2006; 1068: 367-401.
[3]   Body JJ. Rationale for the use of bisphosphonates in osteoblastic and osteolytic bone lesions. Breast 2003; 12: S37-S44.
[4]   Makras P, Papapoulos SE. Medical treatment of hypercalcaemia. Hormones 2009; 8: 83-95.
[5]   Body JJ. Current and future directions in medical therapy: hypercalcemia. Cancer 2000; 88 (Suppl 1): 3054-3058.
[6]   Onuma E, Azuma Y, Saito H, *et al*. Increased renal calcium reabsorption by parathyroid hormone-related protein is a causative factor in the development of humoral hypercalcemia of malignancy refractory to osteoclastic bone resorption inhibitors. Clin Cancer Res 2005; 11: 4198-4203.
[7]   Berenson JR, Lichtenstein A, Porter L, *et al*. Long-term treatment of advanced multiple myeloma patients reduces skeletal events. J Clin Oncol 1998; 16: 593-602.
[8]   Smith MR. Zoledronic acid to prevent skeletal complications in cancer: corroborating the evidence. Cancer Treat Rev 2005; 31 (Suppl 3): 19-25.
[9]   Rosen LS, Gordon D, Kaminski M, *et al*. Long-term efficacy and safety of zoledronic acid compared with pamidronate disodium in the treatment of skeletal complications in patients with advanced multiple myeloma or breast carcinoma: a randomized, double-blind, multicenter, comparative trial. Cancer 2003; 98: 1735-1744.
[10] Lipton A, Theriault RI, Hortobagil GN, *et al*. Pamidronate prevents skeletal complication and is effective palliative treatment in women with breast carcinoma and osteolytic bone metastases: long term follow-up of two randomized, placebo controlled trials. Cancer 2000; 88: 1082-1090.
[11] Guay DR. Ibandronate, an experimental intravenous bisphosphonate for osteoporosis, bone metastases, and hypercalcemia of malignancy. Pharmacotherapy 2006; 26:655-673.
[12] Aapro M, Abrahamsson PA, Body JJ, *et al*. Guidance on the use of bisphosphonates in solid tumours: recommendations of an international expert panel. Ann Oncol 2008; 19: 420-432.
[13] Silverman SL, Landesberg R. Osteonecrosis of the jaw and the role of bisphosphonates: a critical review. Am J Med 2009; 122: S33-S45.
[14] Hoff AO, Toth BB, Altundag K, *et al*. Frequency and risk factors associated with osteonecrosis of the jaw in cancer patients treated with intravenous bisphosphonates. J Bone Miner Res 2008; 23: 826-836.
[15] Ralston SH. Medical management of hypercalcaemia. Br J Clin Pharmacol 1992; 34: 11-20.
[16] LeGrand SB, Leskuski D, Zama I. Narrative review: furosemide for hypercalcemia: an unproven yet common practice. Ann Intern Med 2008; 149: 259-263.

[17]   Zaidi M, Inzerillo AM, Moonga BS, Bevis PJ, Huang CL. Forty years of calcitonin - where are we now ? A tribute to the work of Iain Macintyre, FRS. Bone 2002; 30: 655-663.

[18]   Pondel M. Calcitonin and calcitonin receptors: bone and beyond. Int J Exp Pathol 2000; 81: 405-422.

[19]   Sharma OP. Vitamin D, calcium, and sarcoidosis. Chest 1996; 109: 535-539.

[20]   Wüthrich RP, Martin D, Bilezikian JP. The role of calcimimetics in the treatment of hyperparathyroidism. Eur J Clin Invest 2007; 37: 915-922.

[21]   Khan A, Grey A, Shoback D. Medical management of asymptomatic primary hyperparathyroidism: proceedings of the third international workshop. J Clin Endocrinol Metab 2009; 94: 373-381.

[22]   Peacock M, Bilezikian JP, Klassen PS, Guo MD, Turner SA, Shoback D. Cinacalcet hydrochloride maintains long-term normocalcemia in patients with primary hyper-pathyroidism. J Clin Endocrinol Metab 2005; 90: 135- 141.

[23]   Collins MT, Skarulis MC, Bilezikian JP, Silverberg SJ, Spiegel AM, Marx SJ. Treatment of hypercalcemia secondary to parathyroid carcinoma with a novel calcimimetic agent. J Clin Endocrinol Metab 1998; 83: 1083-1088.

[24]   Lindberg JS, Culleton B, Wong G, *et al.* Cinacalcet HCL, an oral calcimimetic agent for the treatment of secondary hyperparathyroidism in hemodialysis and peritoneal dialysis: a randomized, double-blind, multicenter study. J Am Soc Nephrol 2000; 11: 903-911.

[25]   Kearns AE, Khosla S, Kostenuik PJ. Receptor activator of nuclear factor kappa B ligand and osteoprotegerin regulation of bone remodeling in health and disease. Endocr Rev 2008; 29: 155-192.

[26]   Roodman GD, Dougall WC. RANK ligand as a therapeutic target for bone metastases and multiple myeloma. Cancer Treat Rev 2008; 34: 92-101.

[27]   Clezardin P, Teti A. Bone metastasis: pathogenesis and therapeutic implications. Clin Exp Metastasis 2007; 24: 599-608.

[28]   Burkiewicz JS, Scarpace SL, Bruce SP. Denosumab in osteoporosis and oncology. Ann Pharmacother 2009; 43: 1445-1455.

[29]   Body JJ, Facon T, Coleman RE, *et al.* A study of the biological receptor activator of nuclear factor-kappaB ligand inhibitor, denosumab, in patients with multiple myeloma or bone metastases from breast cancer. Clin Cancer Res 2006; 12: 12211228.

[30]   Crook MK, Guise TA. RANKL: Targeting bone and cancer to treat skeletal complications of malignancy. IBMS Bone Key 2009; 6: 323-338.

[31]   Body J-J, Lipton A, Gralow J, *et al.* Effects of denosumab in patients with bone metastases, with and without previous bisphosphonate exposure. J Bone Miner Res 2009; 25: 440-446.

[32]   Lumachi F, Brunello A, Roma A, Basso U. Cancer-induced hypercalcemia. Anticancer Res 2009; 29:1551-1555.

[33]   Onuma E, Sato K, Saito H, *et al.* Generation of a humanized monoclonal antibody against human parathyroid hormone-related protein and its efficacy against humoral hypercalcemia of malignancy. Anticancer Res 2004; 24: 2665-2673.

[34]   Iguchi H, Aramaki Y, Maruta S, Takiguchi S. Effects of anti-parathyroid hormone-related protein monoclonal antibody and osteoprotegerin on PTHrP-producing tumor-induced cachexia in nude mice. J Bone Miner Metab 2006; 24: 16-19.

[35]   Hall CL, Keller ET. The role of Wnts in bone metastases. Cancer Metastasis Rev 2006; 25: 551-558.

[36]   Voorzanger-Rousselot N, Journe F, Doriath V, Body JJ, Garnero P. Assessment of circulating Dickkopf-1 with a new two-site immunoassay in healthy subjects and women with breast cancer and bone metastases. Calcif Tissue Int 2009; 84: 348-354.

INDEX

A

Acute hypercalcemia (see Chapter 4)	
Addison's disease	21, 25
Adenosin triphosphate (ATP)	190
Advanced Cardiac Life Support (ACLF)	40
Adynamic bone disease (ABD)	14
Aggregation	10
Airway-Breathing-Circulation (ABC)	40
Albumin	3, 20, 32, 38, 39, 45, 46, 47, 51, 53, 88, 95
Albright's calcinosis	11
Alkaline phosphatase (ALP)	23, 56
Aluminum-associated bone disease (AABD)	14
Analytical variation (CVa)	48, 50, 52, 53
Anchoring	10
Anorexia	13, 22, 38
Antidiuretic hormone (ADH)	13
Aryl hydrocarbon receptor-interacting protein (AIP)	24
Asthenia	13

B

Bone alkaline phosphatase (BAP)	50, 51, 56, 57
Bilateral neck exploration (BNE)	79, 80, 81
Bisphosphonates	13, 15, 28, 33, 34, 35, 38, 42, 43, 58, 70, 76 84, 88, 89, 90, 91, 94, 97, 98
Blood pressure	20, 40, 41, 93
BMD see bone mineral density	
Bone mineral density (BMD)	1, 15, 20, 22, 23, 58, 59, 69
Bone morphogenetic proteins (BMPs)	95, 96
Breast cancer	28, 29, 35, 91, 92, 96
Brown tumors	14, 20, 68, 69

C

Calcimimetics	83, 84, 88, 94, 98
Calcitonin	1, 2, 3, 6, 7, 13, 18, 34, 38, 42, 43, 46, 88 91, 93, 94
Calcium sensing receptor (CaSR, CASR)	3, 23, 24, 25, 46, 47, 48, 49, 57, 58, 88, 94
Calciuria	48, 49, 50
Calciphylaxis	15, 16, 39
CASR (CaSR) see calcium sensing receptor	
Central vein pressure (CVP)	40, 41
Chronic kidney disease (CKD)	9, 53
Cinacalcetw	83, 94, 95
c-jun N-terminus kinase (JNK)	31
Competitive immunoassay (IMAs)	54
Computed tomography (CT)	10, 62, 63, 64, 65, 66, 67, 69, 70, 71, 72, 80
Corticosteroids	15, 34
Creatinine clearance	11, 33, 34, 42, 48, 50, 52, 59, 62, 92
Creatinphosphokinase (CPK)	40
CVa see analytical variation	
CT scan see computed tomography	
Cyclin-dependent kinase inhibitor (Kip1)	24

Renal failure	6, 9, 12, 13, 16, 20, 25, 32, 34, 43, 45, 47
	48, 53, 54, 58, 62, 83
Renal stone	10, 68
Renal transplantation	11, 14, 15, 16, 20, 62
RET oncogene	24, 58
Retinoblastoma tumor suppressor (RB) gene	20, 83
Retrotracheal	63, 65, 66
Rhabdomyolysis	6, 13, 25, 51, 62

S

Sarcoidosis	6, 21, 25, 30, 33, 39, 43, 50, 71
Secondary hyperparathyroidism (HPT)	1, 6, 12, 14, 15, 16, 24, 25, 54, 60, 62, 63
	78, 83, 92, 94
Sestamibi	22, 23, 62, 66, 67, 72, 82
SPECT	66, 67, 70
Sovrasaturation	9, 10
Stone disease	11, 68
Surgical treatment of hypercalcemia (see Chapter 7)	

T

TALH see thick ascending limb of Henle's loop	
Tartrate-resistant acid phosphatase (TRAP)	93
TBF-related activation-induced cytokine (TRANCE)	31
99mTc methoxyisobutylisonitrile see 99mTc sestamibi	
99mTc pertechnetate	23
99mTc sestamibi	22, 23, 66, 67, 82
Telopeptide	50, 51, 56, 57, 96
Tertiary hyperparathyroidism	6, 15, 18, 20, 24, 39, 63, 78, 83, 95
Thiazides	6, 8, 18, 21, 43, 59
Thick ascending limb of Henle's loop (TALH)	6, 7, 12
Thyroidectomy	58, 77
Thyrotimic ligament	63, 78, 79
TGF see transforming growth factor	
TNF see tumor necrosis factor	
Total parenteral nutrition (TPN)	13
TRAP see tartrate-resistant acid phosphatase	
Transforming growth factor (TGF)	4, 19, 30, 31, 95, 96
Troponine	40
TRPV5	4, 5, 16, 18
Tumor necrosis factor (TNF)	4, 19, 30, 31, 96

U

Ultra filtrate calcium (UFCa)	7, 19
Ultrasonography (US)	63, 64, 65, 66, 68, 72, 79, 80, 81, 82
Unilateral neck exploration (UNE)	80
Urea nitrogen (sUN)	53
Ureteral stent	11
Uretral calculi	68
Uromether	40
US see ultrasonography	

V

Vitamin D	1, 2, 3, 4, 5, 6, 7, 9, 14, 15. 18, 20, 21, 25, 29
	30, 38, 49, 50, 55, 56, 67, 78, 88, 94, 97

www.ingramcontent.com/pod-product-compliance
Lightning Source LLC
Chambersburg PA
CBHW041719210326
41598CB00007B/713